Hope & Despair

Hope springs eternal in the human breast.

—Alexander Pope

Hope & Despair

How Perceptions of the Future
Shape Human Behavior

Anthony Reading, M.B., B.S., M.P.H., Sc.D.

*Emeritus Professor, Department of Psychiatry and
Behavioral Medicine
University of South Florida
Medical Director, Bay Medical Behavioral Health
Center, Panama City, Florida*

THE JOHNS HOPKINS UNIVERSITY PRESS
Baltimore & London

© 2004 The Johns Hopkins University Press
All rights reserved. Published 2004
Printed in the United States of America on acid-free paper
9 8 7 6 5 4 3 2 1

The Johns Hopkins University Press
2715 North Charles Street
Baltimore, Maryland 21218-4363
www.press.jhu.edu

Library of Congress Cataloging-in-Publication Data
Reading, Anthony.
Hope and despair : how perceptions of the future shape human
behavior / Anthony Reading.
p. ; cm.
Includes bibliographical references and index.
ISBN 0-8018-7948-5 (hardcover : alk. paper)
1. Expectation (Psychology) 2. Hope.
[DNLM: 1. Emotions.   2. Cognition.   3. Mind-Body Relations
(Metaphysics)   4. Thinking. BF 575.H56 R287h 2004]   I. Title.
BF323.E8R32 2004
155.9—dc22
2003026945

A catalog record for this book is available from the British Library.

To

Beth

and

Wendy, Sarah & Greg

and

William & Caroline

Contents

Preface

The way each of us looks at the world is a product of the trajectories our lives have taken. I thought the reader might learn a little about where I am coming from by finding out where I have been. This Preface is thus a kind of personal introduction, to help explain how I became interested in hope and despair—and in the unique way that expectations shape human behavior.

I was born in Sydney, Australia, in 1933. I grew up and went to medical school there and moved to the United States in 1960 to further my education. I have always been an independent thinker, even by Australian standards, a quality that has been both a blessing and a curse over the years. I have also been interested in people for as long as I can remember, in trying to understand what makes them tick, trying to figure out why one person is different from another, and trying to fathom just what it is that makes our species unique. Even in medical school, I was more fascinated by listening to patients talk about their illnesses than by listening to their chests with my stethoscope. These interests led me to the Laboratory of Comparative Behavior at the Johns Hopkins University School of Public Health in Baltimore, where I spent five years learning about the evolutionary biology of behavior. I then thought it would be a good idea to learn more about psychiatry and human behavior, as a way of integrating this newly acquired knowledge with my medical training. So, without any idea of actually *becoming* a psychiatrist, I entered the psychiatry residency program at Johns Hopkins Hospital in 1965. It took about six months for it to dawn on me that this was a fascinating and challenging way of pursuing my long-held interests. Having finally found what I wanted to do as a career, I stayed on the Hopkins faculty for seven years after finishing my training—teaching, seeing patients, and expanding my interest in the relationship between mind and body. I moved to Tampa in 1975 to head the Department of Psychiatry at the University of South Florida College of Medicine, a position I held until 2002. I have remained on the faculty there since, still happy in my career choice and as interested as ever in understanding human behavior.

The year after I completed my psychiatric residency, I received a prize for an essay, "The Nature of Hope." I had become interested in the topic as I puzzled to understand what had gone wrong with the patients I looked after. I was struck by the fact that many of them seemed to have a difficult time predicting where their lives were going—and were thus ill-prepared to deal with whatever befell them. It seemed that they expected either too much or too little of themselves or the world, and ended up being disillusioned and dispirited because of this. They appeared to have gone astray somewhere in their journey along life's highway because of some defect in their ability to generate and maintain realistic hopes about the future. My interest in understanding the impact of expectations on human behavior has only increased over the intervening years, and this book represents a record of where it has taken me.

The past thirty years have been an exciting time to be a student of human behavior. More has been learned about the brain and the mind during this period than ever before. I have thus had the good fortune of witnessing and participating in one of mankind's most remarkable scientific endeavors and have been greatly encouraged by its accomplishments. I have also had the good fortune of having stimulating colleagues, students, patients, and friends who have enriched my experience and furthered my learning. In addition, I have been blessed with more than my share of good luck and with a wonderful family who tolerate my idiosyncrasies and laugh at my jokes. Without these blessings, this book would not have been written, which is why it is dedicated to them.

I would also like to acknowledge the following friends and colleagues for their helpful comments on earlier versions of this manuscript: David Burke, Wendy Burke, Ph.D., Wendy England, Esq., Elisabeth Reading, Ph.D., Sarah Reading, M.D., Kathy Shapiro, Archie Silver, M.D., Irving Weiner, Ph.D., Thomas Wise, M.D., and Jack Zak, M.D. Among the staff at the Johns Hopkins University Press, I would like especially to thank Wendy Harris, for her kindness and perseverance in helping get the book launched, and Anne Whitmore for her diligent editorial assistance.

Introduction

Hope is the pillar that holds up the universe.
—Pliny the Elder

This is a book about hope—and about how its generation and loss shape human behavior. It is about the unique ability that allows our species to generate expectations about the future and base our behavior on them, rather than solely on what is currently happening in our environment. It also explores the remarkable neural mechanisms that enable us to actively shape the future to meet our own designs, rather than have it just repeat the past. Although hope has been the engine that has enabled mankind to develop the complex cultures and civilizations that characterize our species, it is a topic that has largely been ignored by the sciences that study human behavior. It has generally been considered too nebulous a subject to warrant rigorous study and has been relegated instead to the more contemplative realms of philosophy and religion.

One of the reasons science has had such a difficult time coming to grips with hope is that doing so requires understanding how something merely imagined and yet to occur can cause something else to happen. Common sense requires that the cause precede the effect, not come after it. Even more puzzling, not only can something that has not yet happened act as a cause, but so too can something that may never happen, provided that a person *believes* it is likely to happen. The fact that a nonmaterial entity, such as a mere belief, can have such a material effect seems to defy all the laws of physics. How this happens is, of course, still one of the central mysteries of our time—for it is an expression of the complicated relationship that links the mind to the brain.

It is precisely because of this paradox, however, that hope and despair provide such valuable windows for studying the workings of the human mind; for, as we begin to examine the riddle they present, we get a glimpse of the mechanisms that underlie the experience of human consciousness and see the threads that link language, development, and evolution. Hope and despair not only determine much of human behavior; they also help define what makes us so different from the other species. We are the only animals that are able to escape the confines of present time, imagine various scenarios about the future, and base our behavior on the hopes these generate. In order to build these imaginary scenarios, however, the human brain first has to fashion a mental model of the world out of its past experiences. This representational model is what enables us to disengage from the present so that we can recall the past and forecast the future, independent of any current sensory input. One of the main functions of consciousness is to provide a mechanism that allows us to choose between these past, present, and future scenarios and integrate the information they contain. As far as we can tell, other animals do not construct mental models of the universe that enable them to predict what might happen in the future. They are, as a result, limited essentially to the present and to simple expectations of its uninterrupted continuity.

Knowledge about the world has traditionally advanced on two related fronts. One consists of understanding things by taking them apart to see how they work, the so-called reductionistic method, while the other involves putting the pieces together to form composite models, the holistic or systems approach. This book follows the latter course in trying to explain what is so distinctively *human* about human behavior. To do this, it takes information from a number of different fields and tries to shape it into as coherent a whole as possible. Where there are gaps in needed knowledge, plausible inferences have been made to tie the material together. Since much is still unknown about the workings of the human mind, what appear as facts to the author may seem nothing more than speculation to others. As the book itself points out, we are all captives of the belief systems we have built and tend to discount information that does not fit into them.

The focus of this book is thus on the special capacities humans have for processing time, and about the implications this has for improving our understanding of ourselves. Its various chapters illustrate how the mechanisms involved in hope and despair offer a novel way of looking at much of what is puzzling about human nature. They are divided into four sections, each dealing with a different facet of the topic. "The Anatomy of Hope," focuses on our ability to predict the outcomes of our actions and to plan our behavior accordingly. "The Machinery of the Mind" deals with the ways we process sensory information and the implications they have for our understanding of memory, learning, and consciousness. "A Blueprint for Uniqueness" explores the impact that our ability to transcend time has had on our language, emotions, evolution, and individual development. Finally, "The Human Condition" looks at the way our hope-generating abilities shed light on important aspects of our lives, including our social behavior, the relationship between scientific and religious views of the world, and the nature of despair.

Every new book is, in part, a hope-based adventure, for both the writer and the reader. The author's hope is that the ideas expressed here will stimulate others to further explore the unique capacities and limitations of our most extraordinary species.

Part One

The Anatomy of Expectation

Hope is the emotional signature of a special type of expectation. It is a unique amalgam of expectation and desire that our brains fashion to allow us to escape the present and pursue goals that are designed to enhance our future well-being. To make predictions about the future, however, we need a "working model" of the objects and events involved. Much of the genius of our species rests on our ability to construct such mental replicas of the world inside our head, as this is what enables us to imagine and pursue the futures we desire.

CHAPTER 1

The Nature of Hope

When there is no hope, there can be no endeavor.
—Samuel Johnson

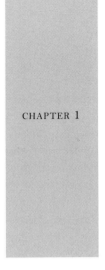

Hope is a uniquely human emotion that energizes us to engage in projects we believe will enhance our future well-being, even though they are of no immediate value to us. Without hope to fuel our dreams and our ambitions, we become captive to whatever is happening in our immediate environment. Without hope's ability to transcend the limits of the present, we lose our sense of ourselves as independent entities, our feeling of mastery, and our sense of purpose. The ability to imagine and anticipate the future is, in fact, a defining aspect of the human condition. Hope gives us a vision that things can be better, rather than just continuing as they have been, an expectation that some desired goal can be attained. It has been the driving force behind all of humanity's great achievements through the ages, the flame that fired the creative energies of our great scientists, inventors, and adventurers. It is also a topic that has fascinated philosophers, theologians, and poets for centuries. But, despite the central role hope plays in shaping human behavior, it has rarely been the subject of serious psychological inquiry. Hope's evanescent nature has made it an elusive target for science, which prefers to deal with more tangible phenomena.[1]

ANTICIPATING THE FUTURE

Hope is an anticipatory emotion, an expectant savoring in our mind of a desired future occurrence that we believe we can help bring about. It differs from ordinary expectation—that things will continue as they have in the past—because it is based on a belief that we can, through our own actions, make something turn out *better* than would otherwise be expected. Most of us base much of our everyday behavior on such hopes, often without realizing how unique this ability is. We go to school in the hope of increasing our knowledge, exercise and take vitamins in the hope of staying healthy, go to work in the hope of receiving a pay check, obey the law in the hope of avoiding punishment, and so on. We also buy lottery tickets, get married, invest in the stock market, quit smoking, buy insurance, work hard, and strive to please, all in hope of increasing future pleasure or decreasing future pain for ourselves or our loved ones.[2]

As far as we can tell, the behavior of all the other species is determined by what their sensory apparatus detects is happening in their current environment—and the associations they make to these perceptions. They have no sense of the future as such and respond entirely to what they see, hear, smell, taste, or feel in their immediate surroundings or to similar changes in their internal state. If they are hungry and what they perceive seems edible, they eat it; if, on the other hand, it looks like it might want to eat them, they run or hide. The other species are unable to generate visions of a future that is independent of their current circumstances. They can, however, learn from past experiences, so the significance of what they perceive can change over time, as also can the way they respond to it. Their behavior is, nonetheless, determined by their current sensory input and the expectations they ordinarily associate with such data, either innately or as the result of experience.

Being able to rise above the demands of the present and create a world that is partly of our own making is one of our crowning evolutionary achievements. The ability to detach ourselves from what is currently going on and mentally roam where our fancy takes us is a distinctly human gift. We are able to conjure up thoughts and images of the future in our mind and act in response to them, our behavior then being determined by what is going on inside our head rather than by what is happening in the world around us. We are thus faced with a choice that no other animal ever has—whether to behave in response to our current circumstances or to our imagined hopes and expectations. The ability to choose which of these to follow provides the basis of our sense of autonomy and free will, as well as our concept of morality.

Hope is a uniquely human amalgam of desire and expectation that motivates individuals to achieve their goals and aspirations. It differs from other types of expectation about the future in that: (a) it is based on what are *believed* to be realistic predictions, and (b) it leads to actions aimed at achieving the desired goals. The aim may be either the attainment of a pleasurable condition or the alleviation of an aversive one, such as the relief of pain or suffering. Because these two outcomes are functionally equivalent, statements about one should be understood to apply also to the other throughout this book.

The word *hope* can be used as either a noun or a verb. Webster's International Dictionary (2nd ed., 1958) defines the noun as "desire accompanied with expectation of obtaining what is desired," while the verb has several meanings, including to desire, expect, wish, and trust. The definition used in this book is based on the noun usage, and is as follows:

> Hope is a pleasurable subjective state that arises when individuals expect that a desired future goal is realistically achievable, and that expectation energizes them to initiate activities they believe will help them attain it.

Hope is thus different from ordinary daydreams, wishes, and desires because these do not generate future-oriented behaviors or elicit its characteristic feelings of anticipatory excitement. Statements like: "I hope I win the lottery," "I hope the train arrives on time," or "I hope the weather will be fine" are really wishes, not hopes in the sense used here. Hope involves more than just expecting some type of pleasurable future. It also involves experiencing a positively expectant emotional state, an increase in energy and motivation, and a targeting of one's behavior to help achieve the desired goal.[3]

Hope entails making a mental appraisal of the likelihood of a desired future state of affairs, based on prior experience and available information. The brain analyzes the ways we might achieve the goal and comes up with predictions about the likely consequences of each of them. Hopes that are generated in this way are great motivating forces—they spur humans to all manner of action and sustain them through periods of trouble and adversity. The more confident we are in our predictions, the greater the amount of energy we have to invest in them, even when they are not correct. Behavior that is designed to bring about a hoped-for future state is referred to in this book as *future-oriented behavior* to differentiate it from behavior that is focused on the present and its immediate extensions.

FUTURE-ORIENTED BEHAVIOR

Future-oriented behavior is the behavioral signature of hope. Such activities as building a house, planting crops, studying for an exam, and investing in the stock market are aimed at achieving a desired goal at some time in the future. Future-oriented individuals, as Zimbardo (1994) observes, "focus primarily on anticipated consequences of possible actions, visualize alternative scenarios associated with different courses of action, and consider liabilities and costs against expected gains." The time frame involved in future-oriented behavior is the out-of-sight, over-the-horizon future, not the one immediately in front of the individual. This distinction is made clear in the French language, which uses different words for the future (*le futur*) and the forthcoming (*l'avenir*), where the latter is simply the extension of the present into the immediate future. St. Paul also observed: "Hope that is seen is not hope: for what a man seeth, why doth he yet hope for?"[4]

Future-oriented behaviors are generally not pleasurable in themselves, for they are aimed at doing things to enhance pleasure or reduce pain at a *later* time. Many are, in fact, sufficiently arduous that most people experience them as *work*—that is, something they have to make themselves do because it is not inherently rewarding. People are usually sustained at such endeavors, however, by savoring the pleasure of their anticipated goal. Future-oriented behavior is thus not a substitute for present-oriented behavior but a complement to it, for the potential benefits of some future-oriented efforts have eventually to be realized as present-time experiences. Choosing between more immediate satisfactions and longer-term goals is, of course an age-old human dilemma. Deferring gratification excessively, as in "all work and no play," is as dysfunctional as not deferring it at all, for such individuals are always on the go, with little time left to savor the fruits of their efforts. Real enjoyment is always experienced in the present; anticipatory pleasures, although agreeable, are simply not as satisfying.[5]

People vary in how well they master the ability to direct their behavior toward the future; it is an acquired skill and has to be learned. Future-oriented behavior is, nonetheless, one of the defining characteristics of modern, industrial societies, even though a number of individuals in them develop little more than a rudimentary capacity for it. Future-oriented activity does not occur to the same extent in less entrepreneurial cultures, which are generally more present-oriented and relatively "timeless" in nature. The capacity for future-oriented behavior evolved over the millennia as our ancestors gradually gained the ability to anticipate the longer-term outcomes of their actions. Although the potential for such behavior is part of our species' common heritage, the degree to which it is expressed depends on the kind of education and cultural heritage to which individuals have been exposed.

Present-oriented individuals generally meet their needs for gratification either by settling for less or by trying to amplify present-oriented sources of pleasure through the increased pursuit of hedonistic activities, including ones involving food, alcohol, drugs, sex, and thrill-seeking. They usually have a difficult time giving up harmful behaviors, since it is the *future* consequences of such activities that are dangerous, not the present ones. They find it particularly hard to quit smoking, for instance, because of the *distant* risk of lung cancer. According to Trivers (1985), the psychologist Paulhan coined the word *presentism* in 1925 to characterize those who experience only the present, and applied the term to babies, most animals, many elderly, and others who seemed to lack the capacity to think beyond the present. Zimbardo (1994) observed that present-orientation was more common among lower-class individuals, who often mix a hedonistic living for the moment with a fatalistic pessimism of never being able to influence the agencies that control their lives. Friedman (1990) found among the poor a similar sense of futility about trying to influence the future and a greater commitment to short-term rewards.

Children do not begin to develop hopes or future-oriented behavior until they acquire a rudimentary capacity for abstract thought and reasoning, usually at about the age of four. Ones who have been abused, neglected, or educationally impoverished often grow up with limited abilities to generate realistic hopes and engage in future-oriented activities. These deficits essentially leave them at the mercy of the present, unable to defer gratification or achieve long-term goals. Such individuals are often unable to inhibit the impulse to respond to current circumstances, even when the consequences of doing so may be quite deleterious to them. Developing into a future-oriented person requires a learned sense of trust in others, along with a set of beliefs about the predictability of people and nature. Zimbardo (1994) says this usually requires growing up in a family and a community with some degree of economic, social, political, and psychological stability, conditions usually absent among the poor, the transient, the abused, and the neglected. He notes that "future-time perspectives are shaped largely through education, certain religious ideologies, family values and models, and the historical accident of being born into a middle-class, urban culture."

Humans are, of course, not the only creatures that engage in behaviors directed toward the future. Many animals have some capacity to anticipate the *immediate* future and foresee the *immediate* consequences of their current actions, but these activities are not future-oriented in the sense used here. Beavers, however, construct dams, salmon swim upstream to spawn, birds fly great distances en route to their migratory destinations, and wasps gather foods to feed larvae they will never see. These relatively fixed behaviors appear to be the result of preprogrammed, instinctual responses to current cues, rather than the product of contemplation about the future. We base *our* future-oriented behavior on conscious consideration of the different options and outcomes we conjure up in our mind's eye. Because of this, human future-oriented behavior is not stereotypically fixed for the species, but differs from one individual to the next.[6]

FAITH

Faith, a variant of hope, is based on belief rather than knowledge. Like hope, it involves positive expectations about the future and generates behavior designed to help make its expectations come true. But the future-oriented behaviors that faith generates, such as prayer and ritual, require the intervention of a deity to achieve their desired outcome, in addition to the individual's own efforts. Faith is essentially based on expectations that are not disprovable—such as the belief that this life's travails are just a prelude to a state of eternal paradise, or that God answers prayers and forgives sinners. While there is a certain logic to hope, albeit one that may often be apparent only to the beholder, faith does not require the same type of rationality to sustain it. Interestingly, although hope is prominent in Judeo-Christian thought and mentioned over 150 times in the Bible, it is not part of the Confucian tradition in Korea and does not appear in the *Analects of Confucius* (Averill, Catlin & Chon, 1990).[7]

Faith's positive beliefs about the future help people endure adversity without succumbing to despair. Like hope, faith sustains true believers by giving them something to look forward to, no matter how difficult their present circumstances. Since hopes are based on experience, new experiences can challenge the assumptions on which they are based—and can reshape them. Faith, however, cannot be as easily shaken by worldly events. It is more difficult to acquire than hope, but also more difficult to lose. Faith can be lost, however, as when a personal tragedy challenges an individual's belief in a beneficent God. The spiritual crisis that results can leave people without a rudder to steer their lives, for the loss of faith can lead to an existential type of despair that questions the very meaning of life. Not all faith is religion-based, however, as people can also have faith in themselves, in human nature, in democracy, or other similar entities.[8]

PASSIVE EXPECTATIONS

Behavior can also be based on passive expectations about the future, rather than on active hopes. These expectations are simply assumptions that the future will essentially resemble the past—that the sun will rise, the rains will fall, and the earth will remain steady under foot. The lives of many current hunter-gatherer societies still revolve around passive expectations about the regularity of the seasons, the harvesting of wild crops, and the migratory patterns of animals. They live, as their ancestors have for centuries, without dreams of things ever having been different from how they now are, or ever becoming different in the future. Unpredictable acts of nature, such as floods, famines, and earthquakes, can severely disrupt such passive expectations, as well as the cultural practices that are based on them.

Passive expectations also occur in more developed cultures. We still base many of our life strategies on such beliefs, often without being aware of their existence until an unexpected disaster occurs and challenges them. Because much of modern civilization has been built on controlling the unpredictable ravages of nature, most of us take for granted that our air and water will be clean, our supply of energy will continue, our homes and schools will be safe, our planes will not crash and our buildings will not fall down. Usually, we only become aware of such passive expectations when something happens to make them no longer seem viable. Unexpected and unanticipated events, such as an untimely death, an economic meltdown, or a terrorist attack, can shake the very foundations of our belief systems.

Different cultures have different sets of assumptions and different expectations about the future. Our sense of shock and disbelief at events depends on the degree to which they challenge our particular set of expectations. A local automobile fatality or a five-year-old child starving in an underdeveloped country hardly get mentioned in the news, for the media focus on reporting the *unexpected*. Passive assumptions that things will keep going on as they have in the past can, however, lead to complacency. Many people continue to pollute the environment and their bodies, just because doing so does not seem to have made much difference in the past.

Passive expectations that everything will just keep going on as before provide a sense of security to conservative individuals, since they generally do not perceive change as an opportunity for future betterment.

OPTIMISM

Optimism is woven into the very fabric of Western society as one of the core ingredients from which its achievements have been fashioned. Columbus, Copernicus, and Newton ushered in new ways of looking at the world by raising the possibility that things could change for the better. Hope triumphed as never before during the sixteenth and seventeenth centuries, as optimistic ideas enlarged the horizons of human endeavor and spurred new waves of artistic and scientific accomplishment. But the path traveled has not always been a smooth one, as many overly optimistic expectations have eventually yielded little but disappointment. Periods of economic and civic optimism have often alternated with ones of economic and civic pessimism, as the Great Depression of the 1930s followed the roaring hopes of the 1920s.

Optimism and pessimism are habitual ways of looking at the future. Optimists hope for the best, no matter what the circumstances, while pessimists always fear for the worst. One is an ingrained tendency to view ambiguous stimuli in a positive light, the other a tendency to view them in a negative one. Whether we "see the glass as half empty or half full" depends on through which of these prisms we view the world. If we do not hope for too much, we will never be disappointed; but we will miss out on opportunities for increasing our well-being. If, on the other hand, we always expect things to turn out for the best, we increase our chances of becoming disappointed and depressed. Since intractable optimism increases errors of commission, and unwavering pessimism errors of omission, individuals with more flexible ways of looking at the future are generally more successful at attaining happy and productive lives.

Studies have shown that optimism and pessimism have far-reaching consequences in achievement at school, at work, and at sports. It is not clear, however, whether a person's attitude can also affect their health and longevity. Although there is anecdotal evidence that supports this popular belief, most physicians remain skeptical about whether the mind can influence the body's response to disease, although they concede it can shape the individual's *experience* of ill health. Optimism is, in fact, one of the main ingredients in the successful physician-patient relationship. Sick people tend to focus their anxieties on the future implications of their symptoms and look to their physicians to provide them with as optimistic a prognosis as possible, that is, a relatively reassuring prediction of what is likely to happen.[9]

The *placebo effect* provides a tangible demonstration of the impact that the mind can have on the experience of illness. Placebos can have a significant effect on reducing pain and other physical symptoms, without necessarily affecting the disorders causing them. One of the most impressive illustrations of the magnitude of the placebo effect was the discovery that sham operations were just as effective in relieving the symptoms of cardiac pain as ones that tied off the internal mammary artery. This latter procedure had gained extremely wide acceptance in the 1950s because it had produced a 90 percent reduction in the frequency of chest pain in cardiac patients, but it rapidly lost favor when the placebo operation produced identical results. The placebo is thought to exert its effect by raising the patient's hopes through heightened suggestion and medical authority, mechanisms that may also explain the effectiveness of a wide variety of nonspecific healing practices and miracle cures.[10]

Despite the skepticism of most scientists, many people believe that hope and faith are critical agents for dealing with the uncertainties of illness, and that they somehow mobilize the body's resources to fight whatever ails them. One of the roles of the healer down through the ages has been to interpret in a hopeful light the impact that the sufferer's symptoms will have on their lives. Spiro (1998) believes that the symbolic meaning of placebo interventions reduces the uncertainty faced by patients who are fearfully concerned about the long-term implications of the symptoms they have been experiencing. He observes that reassurance and positive suggestion from the physician about what the patient can expect bring about relief by raising their hopes and expectations. These ancient healing practices still remain effective in reducing disability and increasing well-being in ways that more current therapies are often unable to reach. The effect of nonspecific interventions can be so great, in fact, that studies designed to determine the effectiveness of new medications are required to take them into account through the use of double blind, placebo-controlled procedures.[11]

HELPLESSNESS

The concept of *learned helplessness* is derived from an experimental model that shows how negative response patterns can be programmed into animals. In this paradigm, dogs are initially trained to expect that moving to the other half of an experimental chamber to escape a mild electric shock will not enable them to avoid the painful experience, as the shock is initially present on both sides of the apparatus. Once this behavior is established, however, the dogs no longer try to escape the shock, even after the electric current on the other side has been turned off. Adversity that *seems* inescapable apparently causes these animals to give up trying to escape, even when this is possible. It is as if they have come to expect that any action on their part would be futile, despite the fact that this is no longer the case. The parallel is obvious—once individuals start avoiding things that they expect will be painful, such avoidances can become a habit if they do not check to see whether their expectations are still accurate.

Helplessness and *hopelessness* are essentially different aspects of the same phenomenon, one being its behavioral guise and the other its emotional one. The research literature deals more with helplessness because it can be defined objectively, whereas hopelessness is a subjective experience that cannot easily be operationalized, especially in other animals. The sense of helplessness arises when individuals feel powerless to bring about desired changes and believe that nothing they do will matter. Sooner or later, they give up trying and quit. The *learned helplessness* model can thus be used to explain the pessimistic outlook and lack of future-oriented behavior that occur in apathy and depression, both of which are discussed further in Chapter 14. Individuals who do not expect that their actions will improve their lot, even when they are not correct in this, tend to down-regulate their autonomic nervous system, cease future-oriented behaviors, and limit themselves to passive ways of responding to the environment. Seligman (1975) maintains that helplessness is at the core of pessimism, but it is not clear which comes first: are people who are relatively helpless at dealing with life's challenges more likely to be pessimistic, or are people who are pessimistic more likely to have trouble dealing with adversities?[12]

FEAR AND ANXIETY

Fear and anxiety are, in some ways, part of the price we pay for being able to predict the future. Unlike hope, these emotions are generated by expectations of harmful events—and lead to escape and avoidance behaviors, rather than productive activities. Fear usually denotes that a specific type of harm is anticipated, such as believing that your plane is going to crash or that you are having a heart attack. Anxiety, on the other hand, is taken to signal a more general state of apprehension, a feeling that any one of a number of potentially undesirable events is likely to occur. The more certain individuals feel that some sort of disaster will happen, the more intense their emotional response and the greater their efforts to escape or avoid the threat. Fear and anxiety are biologically adaptive responses that evolved to help individuals deal with imminent forms of danger. But, as we have become able to escape the confines of the present, they have increasingly come to signal expectations of *future* harm, either real or imagined. Individuals can generate false apprehensions in much the same way they generate false hopes—by filling their future vistas with unrealistic expectations of tragedy and disaster. Unrealistic anxieties about all sorts of possible future harm burden the lives of many people in more entrepreneurial societies and are the basis of a number of psychiatric disorders. The mixture of hope and fear with which we view the future helps shape what we make of it, as well as what it eventually makes of us.[13]

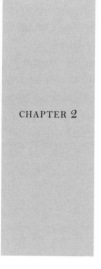

CHAPTER 2

Predicting the Future

> *All our past controls our future.*
> —Alexander Swinburne

The history of civilization is essentially a history of mankind's increasing ability to predict the future. All of our great accomplishments through the ages have been wrought by individuals who first just had an idea in their mind that some as-yet-unheard-of thing could possibly be achieved. As our ancestors began to unravel the lawful regularities of nature, they became increasingly able to anticipate future events and extend the range of things they could master. They learned to control the impact the environment had on them by making clothes, building shelters, taming fire, developing agriculture and, more recently, inventing air conditioning and antibiotics. As magic and superstition gradually gave way to more objective ways of understanding the world, humans became increasingly able to foresee the likely outcomes of their actions and of events in nature. The opening of this window to the future transformed our species by making it possible for us to begin to plan and shape our own destiny.[1]

ORDER AND REGULARITY

Mankind has always been fascinated by the predictable. The daily orbit of the sun, the waxing and waning of the moon, and the changes of the seasons became the first things our ancestors counted on in predicting the future. They were, in fact, so impressed with these recurring acts of nature that they made of them gods, which they worshipped with superstitious rituals and sacrifices. They also afforded special prestige to individuals who claimed to have a gift for seeing into the future. Numerous oracles, prophets, seers, soothsayers, augurs, sorcerers, astrologers, diviners, clairvoyants, and mystics have occupied prominent places in almost every recorded culture. Fortunetellers and psychics flourish to this day in certain communities, and horoscopes are still printed in most daily newspapers. For many, false prophecy is still less frightening than uncertainty.[2]

Our ancestors developed social structures with rules and laws to control human behavior and make our interactions with one another more predictable. These shared ways of understanding the world provide a framework that makes it possible for us to communicate and collaborate with each other. Culture is really little more than a structured set of beliefs and practices that people have superimposed on nature in order to provide an increased level of order and predictability in their day-to-day lives. Different cultures have different beliefs, different rules, different political systems, and different religions, each of which is based on its own set of assumptions about our nature and place in the scheme of things. This is why it is difficult for individuals to change from one cultural or political system to another without first changing their underlying beliefs and assumptions.

We interpret new experiences in terms of previous ones and anticipate what is likely to happen on this basis. We expect people we meet to behave like ones we already know—and we respond to them accordingly, for we have no other way of dealing with them. We initially treat new colleagues, new acquaintances and new persons in authority like ones we have previously known, and unconsciously transfer any left over emotional residues to them. This is the basis of the transference process that psychoanalysts use to explore their patients' relationships with significant figures in the past. Roles like teacher, student, manager, and sales clerk are conventionalized forms of behavior that are sufficiently predictable to allow us to know what to expect without having to get to know each other personally. If we wish to get beyond these stereotypes, to know someone more closely and make contact with them on a personal level, we have to be prepared for the fact that they may no longer fit our previous expectations. We then have to tailor our expectations to match their individual attributes, just as they have to tailor their expectations of us. Knowing someone well enough to be able to predict their behavior with reasonable accuracy is a prerequisite of emotional intimacy.

Predicting what will happen in the future is much like forecasting the weather—it involves making an appraisal of the *likelihood* that certain things will occur, based on prior experience. It depends on understanding the rules and causal chains that link events, so that we can anticipate what is likely to happen in the future. But the future remains veiled in uncertainty until it actually occurs, so the best we can do is predict the *probability* of future occurrences, like a weather announcer, who might forecast a *70 percent chance* of rain. We are able to predict a great many events in such a probabilistic way—like who is *at risk* of having a heart attack or the number of automobile fatalities that will occur over the Memorial Day weekend— but this does not allow us to tell in advance which particular individuals will be affected.

A great many of the everyday decisions we make involve predicting the longer-term costs and benefits of the various choices that confront us. We assess the odds of these, much as gamblers do, and determine how confident we are about our predictions before committing ourselves to action. While this enables us to make predictions for common and repeatable situations with a reasonable degree of accuracy, we have much more difficulty predicting what will happen when a situation is new, its consequences are remote, or its previous outcomes have been erratic. A prediction is like a personal *hypothesis* about how things will turn out, based on the individual's underlying *theory* of what is going on. Just as with scientific theories, it is easier to disprove these personal hypotheses than to prove them by what actually takes place. This is why we base our confidence more on whether we see reasons that our expected outcomes are unlikely to happen, rather than how sure we are that they will occur. The future is always somewhat of a gamble; our task is to develop strategies that maximize the chances of success while minimizing those of harm.[3]

People differ greatly in how confident they need to be before deciding to act. Some are risk averse and need to be virtually certain of the outcome before they start something, while others are willing to take great chances. Decision making involves predicting the value of a desired goal and the likely costs involved in pursuing it. Our brains compute these complex statistical operations almost instantaneously, largely outside our awareness. The process is not foolproof, however, as not all predictions of future well-being turn out. As with electronic computers, the quality of the output depends on the quality of the data on which it is based and the manner in which it is processed. Each of us figures out in our own way, for instance, whether the potential gain exceeds the possible loss when we decide to go to college, get married, invest in the stock market, or visit Las Vegas. Wishful thinking can, however, generate unrealistic hopes that motivate us to engage in behaviors that do not achieve our desired goals.[4]

The amount of confidence we have in our predictions is not directly related to their accuracy; it depends instead on how accurate we *believe* them to be. Our previous levels of success and failure at predicting how things will turn out determine how confident we feel about anticipating what will happen. Self-confident and self-defeating attitudes both tend to be self-fulfilling, however, because they shape how we act and how others respond to us. Successful business leaders often assert that believing in yourself and in what you are doing is an essential ingredient for achievement. Self-confidence is not enough, however, for we also need to have realistic plans for attaining our goals. People who are relatively well off, both psychologically and materially, can usually afford to take greater risks in their lives, as failure will not devastate them, while those who have fewer resources have to be more cautious. Individuals with nothing to lose may take foolish risks, however, generally without giving thought to the consequences.[5]

GENERATING HOPE

The idea that we can shape our own destiny and make our dreams come true is one of the central tenets of Western society. Hopes of fame and fortune have spurred people to prodigious amounts of future-oriented effort—but success is not guaranteed. For every Horatio Alger success, there are also Willy Loman failures who have to settle for lives of unrealized dreams. Those who set their sights too high can burn and crash, like the mythical Icarus who flew too close to the sun. The loftier our aspirations, the more there is to lose. Individuals who have been hurt by lost hopes tend to protect themselves against future disappointment by lowering their sights and dimming their aspirations. People who are hopeful about the future can, however, endure all manner of deprivation and adversity, while those without hope are more easily overwhelmed and defeated.

Hope depends on being able to predict that a desired future is potentially achievable. This involves fashioning a mental model of the variables involved from previously acquired knowledge; the more accurate the model, the more successful the prediction. The birth of modern science in the seventeenth century led to an explosion of knowledge that greatly enhanced our ability to predict natural events. The printing press, public education, and news media then made it possible for ever-increasing numbers of people to obtain the information needed to foresee the longer-term consequences of their own efforts and of events in nature. One of the main functions of education is to provide individuals with a knowledge base that enables them to anticipate and predict what is likely to happen. One's type of knowledge determines the areas in which one can make reliable predictions. Stock brokers thus acquire the knowledge needed to predict the future value of investments, manufacturers the future sales of their products, chefs the results of their recipes, and physicians the course of illnesses. As Merry (1995) points out, individuals with appropriate kinds of knowledge are able to predict and control the outcomes of social and economic systems in ways that can enable them to generate substantial amounts of wealth and power.[6]

A schematic model illustrating the way hope is generated, maintained, and lost is provided in Figure 1. It emphasizes how success and failure along the way toward a desired goal provide feedback that either increases or decreases the amount of hope experienced. Individuals usually have a number of long- and short-range goals, with success in some helping offset failure in others, a balance that helps them keep their hopes alive during temporary setbacks. But if they eventually run out of possibilities for attaining the things they desire, at least as they see it, they lose all hope—and depression ensues. People whose behavior has been based primarily on achieving future goals no longer have anything left to motivate or guide them. Clinical depression is like a time-out during which individuals who are unable to generate hope are left to make the most they can out of their present circumstances.[7]

The extent to which our expectations motivate and energize us is proportional to the amount of hope they generate. This, in turn, depends on how confident we are that our expected good fortune will come to pass and on how much pleasure we anticipate it will bring. Our overall sense of hopefulness is a function of the amount by which our total positive expectations exceeds our total negative ones at any given time. At one extreme, manic individuals get so buoyed up by their grandiose expectations that they can keep going for days on end without feeling a need to stop to eat or sleep, while at the other extreme, severely depressed ones retreat into a state of behavioral withdrawal and inactivity. How we see the future determines much of what we do.

Anticipated pleasures generate positive emotional states that mimic their corresponding real-life experiences. Being able to savor the emo-

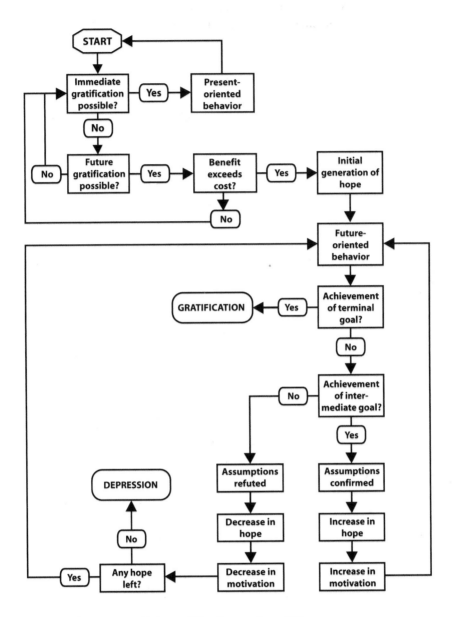

Figure 1. The Generation of Hope

tional component of what we picture in our imagination enables us to evaluate just how gratifying a particular future would be. Fantasized pleasures are not as satisfying as real ones, however, in the same way that low-fat, low-calorie foods don't taste like the genuine articles. But imagined enjoyment can be a source of support that helps sustain people through difficult times. Individuals who are hungry or overworked can, for instance, dream about having a feast or taking a vacation. The pleasurable feelings associated with hope are, however, much stronger than those associated with mere fantasy, for hope is based on a *believable* expectation that the desired future will actually happen.[8]

The lure of fantasy satisfactions entraps some people so completely in thoughts of the future that they end up neglecting the present. For them, deferring gratification becomes a habit in itself. They live in a world of planning great things that never eventuate, saving frugally rather than buying things that would give them pleasure, or sacrificing themselves endlessly in hope of one day being appreciated. Too much future-oriented behavior can be as hazardous to one's health as too little, for all real gratification takes place in the present. Our future-oriented hopes must one day be realized in a tangible way if they are to enhance our sense of pleasure and well-being—for the future one day becomes the present.

EXPECTANCY

A great deal of our everyday behavior is shaped by expectations, by assumptions both conscious and unconscious of what follows what. Passive expectations of the more immediate outcomes of our own actions and of events around us are not, however, associated with hope. This simple type of expectation shapes much of what we do and how we respond to events around us and is based on the associations our brains make from what we have previously experienced. The short-range predications that guide many of our moment-to-moment behaviors differ, however, from the longer-range computations required to generate hope. Their passive expectations are based on assumptions that the future will be much like the past, whereas hope is predicated on the belief that the future can be different from the past.[9]

Expectancy is a construct that has been widely used to study and understand human behavior. Expectancy-value theories that combine expectations of outcomes with expectations of their value, either good or bad, figure prominently in studies of human motivation. As Zaleski (1994) and Calne (1999) point out, all human motivation is future-oriented, since it refs to striving for anticipated goals that are not yet present. Although *motives* are similar to *hopes* in that they both generate goal-oriented behaviors, they differ from them in that they do not generate anticipatory emotional reactions, have only general goals (e.g., to become wealthy), and do not involve specific plans or expectations of actual achievement. Motives and drives are psychological constructs used to explain why individuals make the behavioral choices they do, even when they are not themselves aware of the reasons.[10]

People who are able to use expectations to plan their behavior and achieve goals they set for themselves generally feel more in control of their lives than those who do not have the same sense of personal agency. Rotter (1966) contrasts people who believe everything is due to passive expectations, such as luck, fate, or powerful others, with ones who see themselves as able to shape their own futures. He portrays individuals who have an *external* locus of control as being more passive and fatalistic, and those who have an *internal* locus of control as more focused on achieving their desires. Bandura's (1997) theory of self-efficacy similarly asserts that people who expect more of their own capabilities are more likely to be motivated to solve problems they encounter and plan for the future. A great deal of psychopathology is, however, related to errors in expectancy, whether about one's own abilities, the behavior of others, or the environment. Phobias, for instance, are due to expectancies that harm will occur if the feared object is contacted, while paranoid individuals expect that others are plotting to hurt them. Such negative expectancies unfortunately often lead to behaviors that tend to perpetuate them.

DEALING WITH UNCERTAINTY

The best we can do at piercing the veil that hides the future from us is to reduce some of its inherent uncertainty, since this can never be entirely eliminated. As a result, every prediction that we make will be limited in some way. The more complex the subject and the more distant the time frame, the less accurate our predictions are likely to be. In theory at least, if we knew everything there was to be known about something, we could predict its future with total accuracy, because deterministic systems are perfectly predictable once all of their initial conditions and operating rules are specified. Some things are essentially unpredictable, however, because their inherent complexity or chaotic nature makes it impossible to identify all of the determining factors. These inevitable uncertainties limit our abilities in fields ranging from subatomic physics to galaxial cosmology, and even thwart our efforts to know what will happen to the economy and the environment over time. They also frustrate us in our everyday decisions about how to invest our energies and resources to secure a better tomorrow for ourselves and our families.[11]

We make predictions by building models that link the variables we believe to be relevant and specifying, as best we can, the rules that govern their interactions. The models do not have to be physical replicas of the systems involved but can be diagrams, sketches, mathematical equations, computer simulations, or even verbal theories, provided that the information they contain corresponds well enough with the information in the system being modeled. They can also be the models our brains construct to enable us to understand the world and make projections about the future. A model's effectiveness as a predicting device depends, of course, on the extent to which it captures the critical variables and relationships. Because these are often difficult to specify with certainty, most models contain a number of assumptions, some of which may be quite speculative. As a result, the best that even the most sophisticated simulations can usually do is specify a range of possible outcomes and estimate the statistical odds that each of them will occur. Brand (1999) suggests, along the same lines, that the most effective strategy in everyday life is to try to predict a range of possible eventualities and make contingency plans to deal with each of them so we can be prepared for whatever befalls us.[12]

Some models are too general to be used for prediction, even though they can provide explanations of how things work. Darwin's theory of natural selection, for instance, is a model that can explain the evolution of the various species but cannot predict it—for too many variables are involved to be enumerated with any degree of accuracy. Masterpasqua and Perna (1997) point out that our individual life courses provide another example of complex systems that are understandable but not predictable—for, although they are determined by lawful processes, these interact in ways that are too complex for us to specify with precision. Trefil (1997) believes, for the same reasons, that even though our understanding of the brain may eventually enable us to explain many of our activities, it is unlikely that it will ever be sufficient to predict them. He observes that we would first have to know where every neuron was and how it was connected to all of the others in order to predict such emergent functions as consciousness and self-awareness.

Thus, although events may be caused by antecedent events, they are not necessarily predictable—that is, they are determined, but not necessarily determinable. *Accident* is the name we give to an adverse event that was considered not predictable, something that was not expected to happen, like the crash of the Concorde or the sinking of the Titanic. While the *fact* that automobile accidents or natural disasters will happen is predictable, the circumstances of particular accidents or disasters are not. We can, however, retrospectively examine the events that led up to such incidents to understand what happened and use this information to help prevent or moderate the effects of similar occurrences in the future. Untoward medical outcomes also involve issues of predictability. Adverse incidents that are predictable are considered to be preventable and thus, when they occur, are regarded as evidence of negligence, whereas those perceived as unpredictable are not. We are, in fact, not held responsible in the eyes of the law for acts whose untoward outcomes could not to a reasonable degree have been foreseen.[13]

Good fortune can also be unpredictable when caused by indeterminable factors. We usually ascribe this to luck or chance, even though good accidents are no more capricious than bad ones. The ancients used to believe that such events were determined by fate or some other immaterial force, for everything had to have a definable cause. No matter how much understanding we have, emergent and unforeseen events will occur and will shape how things turn out in ways that we cannot possibly predict, even when we can see them in hindsight as inevitable reactions to what was going on. The *retrospectoscope* is great for explaining how something happened after the fact, but it is of little use in predicting how it will happen next time. Unpredictable events bring responses of surprise and disbelief, the degree of surprise being a fairly accurate measure of how unexpected they were. Reactions of surprise occur as much with unanticipated good fortune as with bad, as much on hearing you have won the lottery as on learning that your house has burned down. Shackle (1962) notes, "It is only a man who feels very sure of a given outcome who can be greatly surprised by its non-occurrence."[14]

CHAPTER 3

The Internal Representation of the External World

No man's knowledge here can go beyond his experience.
—John Locke

The fact that we are able to think about objects and events that are not physically present indicates that we have some type of mental representation of them inside our head. We build mental models of the universe out of our experiences and later manipulate them to create our own private realities. We all live in two worlds: an external one of the objects and events we experience and an internal one of the concepts and abstractions we create from them. The process is so unobtrusive that most of us do not realize that our brains have constructed these mental replicas—we simply assume the world inside our head is the same as the one outside it. We believe that our ideas about the universe and how it works are reflections of external reality, rather than of the models we have constructed to represent it. We build and modify our internal worlds from our sensory experiences and from what we make of them—and they are limited because of this. Everything we encounter is not simply recorded in memory like a home movie but instead is filtered, analyzed, and processed to build representations that can be adjusted in response to new information.[1]

Our internal models are what enable us to make generalizations, infer relationships, have beliefs, and fashion thoughts and images not cued by current circumstances. They are also what makes it possible for us to imagine the future, generate predictions of what is likely to happen, and use these to achieve things we desire. The more accurately our models represent the external world, the more likely we are to realize our aspirations. The nature of our internal representations and the manner in which they are encoded by the brain are, however, only speculative, as no one has yet identified how they actually function. Their existence is, nonetheless, well supported by the available data. Johnson-Laird (1983) observes that "it is now plausible to suppose that mental models play a central and unifying role in representing objects, states of affairs, sequences of events, the way the world is, and the social and psychological actions of daily life." He notes that understanding something means being able to develop a working model of it—i.e., knowing how its components relate to each other and how it relates to other entities. Fortunately, the models we make do not have to be entirely accurate in order to be useful; they just need to be accurate enough for the purpose at hand.[2]

MENTAL REPRESENTATIONS

The human brain can represent external objects and events in two distinct ways. *Sensory representations* are neural engrams that represent the objects and events we encounter, based on input from our various sensory receptors. They constitute encodings of particular sensory experiences, such as the face of a friend or the image of a particular building, static replicas of specific objects and events. Like photographs and maps, they do not themselves portray information about the time of their occurrence or their relationships with other entities, since these qualities are *inferred* rather than *experienced*. The neural patterns that capture these sensory representations are the basis of recognition memory and associative learning, phenomena in which current sensory input either resembles or is linked to a previously encoded configuration. *Symbolic representations*, on the other hand, are engrams that encode words, numbers, and abstract images, as well as the relationships that link objects and events together. They include concepts like *gravity* and *health*, and categories like *house* and *tree*, as well as our sense of time and of self. Because the symbolic system deals with abstract information and inferences, rather than concrete events, it is able to indicate the relationships between its representational entities—a feat the simpler sensory system is not able to accomplish. These include the causal relationships and rules that link representational elements to form a model of the individual's world. Symbolic representations enable us to *understand* what has happened to us, create personal belief systems, and forecast the future.[3]

The ability to create abstract models that depict the rules governing the interactions between the objects and events we experience is, as far as we can tell, a defining feature of the human nervous system. Although a number of other species seem to have a form of mental representation for familiar surroundings and for individuals in their own group, these are isolated capacities that do not constitute a representational *system*. The use of twigs by chimpanzees to fish for termites, the way sea otters carry rocks from the sea bottom to the surface to crack open hard crabs, and the wiggle dance of bees communicating the location of nectar all seem to indicate the presence of specific representational abilities. Humans are unique, however, in being able to develop a representational system that encodes the symbols and abstractions that constitute the basis of language and forethought. Our representational systems are not monolithic but, rather, consist of a loosely connected number of subsystems, each of which is made up of knowledge in a domain of importance to the particular individual. People vary greatly in the nature and complexity of their knowledge domains—only some of us know how to program a computer, build an igloo, or do heart surgery. The model of the world that we construct is thus like a confederation of linked submodels, with each being sufficient to allow prediction in its own area of knowledge but not in others.[4]

The concept of mental representation has become a central tenet of the field of cognitive psychology. Crook (1980) notes, "Representative processes are at the root of man's capacity to deal with the abstract qualities of objects and events, his ability to deal with the possible or conceivable, the ideal as well as the actual, the intangible along with the tangible, the absent as well as the present object or event, with fantasy and with reality." As Paivio (1986) observes: "The problem of how we represent information mentally and how we use that information to interact with the world in adaptive ways is an old and persistent one. Our distant ancestors must have wondered about it long before they knew how to represent information on the walls of caves or on wax tablets; and we still wonder, though we know how to represent information in computers and use it with lightning speed. The problem persists because it is extraordinarily difficult, perhaps the most difficult one in all of science. It is essentially a question of the nature of knowledge and of thought, and all that these imply in terms of observable behavior, brain activity, developmental origins, environmental effects, and so on."

The information we use to construct our mental model has to be fed into our nervous system in an orderly and intelligible fashion if it is to be effectively incorporated, since little can be learned from overwhelming chaos or complexity. The first world that gets programmed is the world of the infant—mother, breast, bottle, light, noise, faces, voices, and so on. As youngsters get exposed to an ever-widening range of stimuli and interactions, the behavioral repertoires that enable them to master their small worlds become increasingly elaborate. Growing children keep applying the model they have so far developed to an ever-larger universe, adding to it and modifying it as new experiences accumulate. The developing youngster's representations coalesce into generalizations whose accuracy depends on the nature of the experiences on which they are based and the inferences that have been made from them. Children who are raised by unloving, inconsistent, or negligent parents, for instance, often grow up with distorted models of themselves and of the way people relate to each other. Schools, churches, and peer groups also help shape our mental models, so that in well-knit communities the ideas and beliefs of different individuals have a great deal in common. Divergent cultural groups share fewer assumptions and often misunderstand each other because of this disparity, which is one of the reasons why differences in class, ethnicity, and family background are such effective barriers to social integration.[5]

We construct our mental models of the universe piece by piece from what we encounter and how we experience it. The largely unconscious process by which this occurs involves searching for patterns in what we experience, for similarities and differences between the various events we encounter. The object is to build a model whose components are as compatible as possible, both with each other and with the external world. This ideal is never fully achieved, however, as the process is like trying to assemble a gigantic jig-saw puzzle without having all the pieces. We may find several components that seem to fit together but then have trouble seeing where they articulate into the larger scheme of things. The more we make mistakes in our assumptions about how the initial pieces fit together, the more difficult it is to link the parts that contain these errors to other sections of the puzzle. As a result, the models that we build usually contain significant areas of internal discord, which can become sources of mental conflict when they lead to incompatible goals and expectations.[6]

If we encounter facts that do not fit into the model we have so far developed, we have to give up some of our current beliefs, reject the new information, or compartmentalize it in our minds so that it does not affect our current belief system. The latter two options lead, however, to a distorted view of the world that can impair our ability to predict the future correctly. The deeper and more fundamentally held our views, the more difficult it is to change our underlying models, even when new information fits the facts better. Learning involves both assimilating new information that is compatible with our current beliefs and adjusting our beliefs to accommodate the new data when it is incompatible (Piaget & Inhelder, 1969). Unlearning something we have previously learned is much more difficult than learning something new, especially if it means having to modify an existing model. This may explain why we generally like to read books that confirm our beliefs and associate with people who share our views.

Kuhn (1970) points out that our knowledge base does not grow solely by the simple accretion of new facts but occasionally undergoes fundamental changes in the underlying models on which it rests, which he calls paradigms. This occurs when new facts accumulate that do not fit into the existing model, with the result that a more all-encompassing paradigm needs to be developed. He notes that radically new ideas have always been met with resistance by the establishment, and he quotes Darwin's statement at the end of *On the Origin of Species:* "Although I am fully convinced of the truth of the views given in this volume, I by no means expect to convince experienced naturalists whose minds are stocked with a multitude of facts all viewed, during a long course of years, from a point of view directly opposite to mine. But I look with confidence to the future, to young and rising naturalists, who will be able to view both sides of the question with impartiality." Calvin (1996) notes Haldane's comment on the topic: "The four stages of acceptance of a scientific theory are: (1) this is worthless nonsense, (2) this is an interesting but perverse point of view, (3) this is true, but quite unimportant, (4) I always said so."[7]

Thinking involves the creation and manipulation of mental representations of objects and events that do not need to be present in the current environment. It is a process that helps us make sense out of what happens to us and decide what to do. Rational decision making is based on considering the likely consequences of alternative courses of action, based on estimating the probability of benefit and harm associated with each of them. We choose a given path because it is likely either to maximize personal pleasure or benefit those we care about. All of the potential outcomes are, however, merely predictions whose accuracy depends on having an effective working model of whatever is being considered. The options we eventually select integrate information from the two worlds in which we live—the material one we share with everyone else and the private, mental one that we create to give meaning to what we experience.[8]

PERSONAL CONSTRUCTS

We build our model out of a series of personal constructs that we develop to catalogue and organize our experiences, and we then use these as a framework for trying to understand the other objects and events we encounter. Kelly (1955) called these templates *constructs* because they represent the way we *construe* the world. He pointed out that it is how we construe events, what each of us makes of what happens to us, that determines our behavior, not the events themselves. We try to understand unfamiliar objects and events in terms of constructs with which we are already familiar. If the analogy between them is only superficial, the fit may not be good, but a poor fit may be better than no fit at all in trying to make sense of the world. Our lives would otherwise consist largely of a series of unrelated events, much as the world appears to the newborn and the severely demented person. Since we are able to incorporate new information into our models only in terms of constructs with which we are already familiar, we are limited in what we can imagine and understand by what we already believe. As Haldane (1940) once remarked, "the universe is not only queerer than we suppose, but may be even queerer than we can suppose."[9]

Constructs are organized into hierarchical systems that become more abstract with each increasing level of organization. Some of this can be seen in the associations we have to the names of various entities—the things that first come to mind in connection with them. Typical associations to the word *apple*, for instance, may include *orange, fruit, red, core, eat, pie, sauce, tree,* and *orchard,* indicating the way different constructs are linked in the brain. We also develop constructs about the nature of the relationships between different entities, including temporal ones like *earlier* and *later, faster* and *slower,* and spatial ones like *higher* and *lower, larger* and *smaller.* The various kinds of relationships that we use to describe how entities are connected are *constructs* that we infer but do not directly experience. The structural, functional, and causal relationships that link entities in our models mirror the ones we perceive in the external world, since they are both created in the brain. Mathematics and geometry, for instance, entail functional relationships, such as the one between the radius and circumference of a circle. Music is an example of a temporal pattern in which each succeeding note is structurally, but not causally, related to the preceding one. On the other hand, matches and fire, infection and fever, loss and sadness involve causal relationships. The progressive discovery over the millennia of the relationships between entities in the natural world is what the growth of knowledge has been all about.[10]

THE ASSUMPTIVE WORLD

Our representational models include a number of beliefs and assumptions about ourselves and the world that shape our perceptions and guide our behavior. The totality of these personal beliefs, many of which are not fully conscious, may be conveniently termed our *assumptive world*. This refers to an organized set of interacting values, expectations, and images, many of which are shaped by the myths and folkways of the culture into which we are born. The assumptive worlds that we create range from the simple and poorly differentiated to the complex and highly structured, depending on our experience, intellect, and education. The models we create may also *mis*represent the world to greater or lesser degrees, leading us to harbor any number of false beliefs. The more erroneous our assumptions, the less accurate are the plans and expectations we base on them. The assumptive worlds of people with psychotic disorders, for instance, are based so extensively on false beliefs that these individuals are said to be "out of touch with reality." Untreated, they live in their own private worlds, unable to manage their affairs or communicate effectively with others.[11]

The members of a family, a group, or a community who share an erroneous assumptive world are able to communicate and understand each other, even though they may have a difficult time relating to outsiders. Shared belief systems form part of the glue that binds people together, even when they are based on flawed or unrealistic assumptions. People who believe in alien abductions or fanciful conspiracy theories find validation and comfort in being able to communicate and connect with one another, even though these beliefs may otherwise mislead them. Different groups and different cultures develop different ways of understanding the world— and a great deal of human blood has been spilled as a result. While other animals fight over mates or territory, humans tend to fight over ideologies. The beliefs that various people have that their way of life or religion is specially blessed or entirely correct cannot all be true. The fact that humans are so willing to lay down their lives for their convictions is, however, an indication of how vital these conceptual schemes are—and how important it is for people to believe that *their* world view is the correct one.

Every culture builds its own explanatory model of the universe, based on the particular truths that are of salience to it. Cultures tend to converge and become more alike over time, however, as knowledge and understanding become disseminated through trade, migration, and warfare. Science also tends to foster convergence, since its methods are designed to be free of personal and social bias. The large systems of knowledge that science has created, like chemistry, biology, and psychology, do not fit well together, however, which is why they remain separate disciplines. The fact that we compartmentalize knowledge into these discrete realms is due to our limited understanding of the universe—and possibly our limited capacity for understanding it. Even science ends up with a series of partial models that are useful for predicting within particular spheres, but not outside of them.

THE SELF

We also develop a mental representation of our own selves—who we are, what we look like, and what we stand for. This mental model of our self encodes our ideas about our distinctive interests, tastes, aversions, talents, proclivities, and the like, as well as our evaluations of our own competences and self-worth, or lack thereof. We develop a mental representation of our self as an entity in time and space, a notion of our own unique identity, in the same way we develop conceptual models of other people. Our sense of self provides a feeling of coherence between our past and our expected future, as captured in the stories we carry with us about who we are, where we have been, and what we anticipate doing. Patients with Alzheimer's disease lose this sense of self and personal identity when they are no longer able to remember who they once were.[12]

One of the first tasks that developing infants master is differentiating themselves from the rest of their universe. They learn early on to recognize that their arms and legs are connected to them and that other objects are not. Their ideas of *self* gradually expand over time to include a sense of their own unique mental and physical characteristics. Many of the identity problems that characterize the transition from adolescence to adulthood involve differentiating what are truly our own ideas, beliefs, and values from those that we have taken in from others. Individuals who have a sound sense of personal identity tend to have a well-functioning model of the world, for *self* and *non-self* are essentially reciprocal constructs, opposite sides of the same representational coin. The emphasis on individual identity that characterizes much of Western society can lead, however, to an almost pathological preoccupation with self and self-interest. Many non-Western cultures emphasize group identity and fulfillment more than individual achievement.

As part of our sense of self, we come to believe that our lives should have a purpose and meaning beyond our own self-interest and existence. It seems that we need to feel that we are a part of something larger than ourselves and have something outside of our self that is important to us. This is what tends to make us feel that life is worth living and what we do matters. While it is not entirely clear what gives rise to the sense of meaning in our lives, it is an aspect of the assumptive world we create. When faced with the unimaginable vastness of the universe, we like to think that everything has a reason for being the way it is, ourselves included, for the possibility that life is completely pointless is too frightening to contemplate. Meaning and purpose are, however, qualities we bestow on events in order to make the world seem more understandable, not inherent properties of the things we experience.[13]

The ultimate differentiation of self involves taking responsibility for one's own actions, rather than blaming others for what happens. Becoming a mature and self-actualized person is, in fact, based on taking ownership of one's own beliefs and behavior. Although this type of authenticity allows individuals to take credit for what they accomplish, it also requires them to own up to their shortcomings, no matter how disconcerting this may be. The fundamental value of a more accurate mental representation of one's *self* is that it provides a more realistic basis for self-actualization and for predicting how best to achieve one's goals. Depersonalization is a state in which people experience their own self as strange and unreal. Such a dissolution of the sense of one's own identity can occur under conditions of extreme stress, under the influence of certain drugs, and in certain mental disorders.[14]

TRUTH AND FALSITY

The mental models we construct can never fully apprehend reality, because our systems of knowledge and understanding are all built on initial beliefs that cannot themselves be proven. We have to take something for granted before we can understand something else, to start with an initial point of reference that we accept implicitly before we can institute logical operations. The brain cannot create new conceptual elements *de novo;* the only way it creates new mental constructs is by rearranging and recombining elements from older ones. Creativity largely involves producing something novel through the rearrangement of already-known constituents, first in the mind and then later in the world. We reason by analogy and use metaphors—as when we conceive of the body as some sort of machine or of electrons orbiting an atomic nucleus as being like planets orbiting the sun—and see how well these models fit. All of the facts and certainties we know are only true within arbitrary frameworks that are themselves not provable. It is not possible, for instance, to prove that a belief is true, because our neuronal structures are only able to detect that something is false.[15]

We are all scientists in our own way, trying to make sense out of the world with our remarkable information-processing capabilities. One of the differences between scientific and ordinary human reasoning, however, is that science devises experiments to test its theories, whereas everyday understanding depends on *experiments of nature* to confirm its beliefs. A great deal of our thinking involves developing and applying rules in order to understand different aspects of the world, predict what is likely to happen, and make choices between the options that confront us. The rules we develop are like theories that articulate perceived causal relationships between things we have experienced. These ideas are then either supported or refuted by the subsequent events we experience. Because our theories cannot be directly confirmed, we test them by assessing the validity of the predictions that we base on them. Our predictions are really nothing more than hypotheses about a future state of affairs, and they are either validated or invalidated by what eventually takes place.[16]

Despite the fact that we are only able to approach the truth by systematically identifying what is untrue, we have assembled an impressive edifice of knowledge over the millennia through a process of ever-closer approximations. Theories that are so self-contained as to prevent the construction of hypotheses that might invalidate them are not considered to be true scientific theories. Ideas that are based on belief rather than on empiric data, no matter how useful they may be, are not subject to refutation by additional experience. The underlying theories of id, ego, and superego on which much psychoanalytic thought is based are examples of assumptions that have to be accepted or rejected implicitly, as there is no way of proving or disproving their existence. Although beliefs based on faith may help structure and give meaning to our lives, they are of little help in predicting how the future will turn out.[17]

Part Two

The Machinery of the Mind

Over the millennia, the human brain has developed highly sophisticated capabilities that enable it to process information in ways not found in any other species. We humans are able to construct mental models that let us recall the past and predict the future. We also possess a form of consciousness that allows us to experience a sense of self and an awareness of time. Our emotions provide us with information about the value of the objects we perceive, the relationships we enter, and the plans we make to enhance our future well-being.

CHAPTER 4

The Processing of Information

> *"In nature's infinite book of secrecy, a little can I read."*
> —The Soothsayer, *Antony and Cleopatra,*
> William Shakespeare

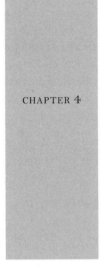The human brain and mind are simply two facets of an amazing information-processing system that has been molded by evolution over the millennia. They function as one to process information from our internal and external environments in such a way that our responses are as appropriate and adaptive as possible. *Mind* and *brain* are, however, not separate entities that exist independently of each other—they are merely different aspects of the remarkable central nervous system with which we have been endowed. We have created constructs of them as separate to help us understand the complex processes involved, viewing one as concerned with structure and the other with function. *Mind* is an abstraction that describes what the *brain* does, in much the same way that the process called digestion describes what the stomach does. The mind is not a separate entity located somewhere in our head or an ethereal force that guides our behavior. The duality between mind and body which Descartes described three centuries ago now serves mainly to hinder our understanding of their function.[1]

MIND AND BRAIN

Mind is a concept that refers to a collection of subjective phenomena that enable us to experience conscious thoughts and feelings. It is used to explain our sense of having a self that makes decisions and determines how we behave. The *brain*, on the other hand, is a tangible, material object that obeys the laws of physics and chemistry. All of our thoughts and feelings are represented in it by physical and chemical changes that activate and shape our lives. Our loftiest hopes, our most fanciful dreams, and our worst nightmares all have biochemical representations somewhere within its fragile tissues.[2]

The human brain is the most complex and highly organized structure in the known universe. It is composed of some 100 billion neurons, each with about a thousand synapses that connect it to other neurons and to the body's sensory and motor systems. It has been estimated that if all the connections between these nerve cells were placed end to end, they would stretch about one hundred thousand miles. Almost half of the neurons reside in the cerebral cortex, the brain's outermost layer, where they fire from 40 to 1,000 times per second during the entire time we are awake. This three-millimeter-thick mantle of tissue, which contains the very essence of our humanity, would cover an area less than three square feet if it were laid out flat. Even so, it is four times larger than the comparable brain region in the chimpanzee. One measure of how tirelessly the human brain functions is that it consumes twenty percent of our daily energy requirements—even though it makes up only two percent of our total weight.[3]

Because we understand things only in terms of other entities with which we are already familiar, we usually conceptualize the brain as a telephone exchange or a computer. But these models fall far short of explaining the intricacies of its internal workings. Computers are essentially logic machines that do not understand the meaning or significance of the symbols they are programmed to use. They do not have the sensory and emotional inputs that color our mental lives or the subjective experiences that characterize consciousness. While they can be programmed to mimic some of the operations of the brain, they are not able to simulate the subjective functions of the mind, such as appreciating beauty, exhibiting empathy, or having a sense of oneself as an entity in time and space. As Dennett (1996) points out, while computers can be programmed to process symbolic information and read texts, they do not *understand* what they read. Information in the brain is not like information in a computer, as the former has a meaning shaped by the individual's past experience and social environment.[4]

The human brain is endowed with two interconnected systems for processing, assessing, storing, retrieving, and responding to information. The *sensory information system* gives real-time information about environmental and physiological events that activate our various sensory receptors. This phenomenon is a fundamental biologic endowment we share with the rest of the animal world. The *symbolic information system* is a product of human development and enables us to process the meaning of language and other abstract symbols. It can access information recalled from the past or imagined about the future—in ways that distinguish our mental capacities from those of other species. While the sensory system is able to capture aspects of our own experience of the world, the symbolic one enables us to learn what others have experienced, as communicated to us through spoken and written language. The sounds and sights that convey such verbal transactions, although initially perceived by the sensory system, differ from other perceptual experiences in that they have to be decoded to access the information they contain. When we are not able to do this, as on overhearing an unfamiliar language being spoken, the information contained is simply not available. Language enables our symbolic system to supplement our sensory one in ways that exponentially increase our knowledge and understanding of the world.[5]

THE SENSORY INFORMATION SYSTEM

The body is endowed with a large number of sensory receptors that provide information about the current state of its external environment and its internal milieu. Data from these different sources are relayed to the brain, where they are integrated and interpreted in order to generate adaptive physiological and behavioral responses. Both the incoming information and the outgoing responses are represented in the brain by unique patterns of neuronal firing. These neuronal firing patterns are then *remembered*, so that stimuli that produce comparable firing patterns in the future can be recognized as being similar. These neuronal patterns can be modified by subsequent experience, enabling individuals to change how they respond to a given stimulus, a process that constitutes the neural basis of learning.[6]

The sensory system records the salient aspects of the various objects and events we experience and stores them as neurochemical engrams that allow them to be recognized at a later time. We are largely unaware that our brain is being constantly bombarded with sensory input about our surroundings from our senses of vision, hearing, touch, taste, and smell, as well as information about the workings of our internal organs. Most of the input about the body's internal state of affairs is, in fact, processed automatically by built-in self-regulating mechanisms that do not intrude into consciousness. We usually become aware of our bodily functions only when illness or injury disrupts their normal operation. A great deal of the input from the external environment is also processed outside of awareness, leaving us free to focus our attention on a given task without being distracted. Much of the brain's regulatory apparatus is, in fact, devoted to inhibiting neural responses that are not pertinent to the task at hand. These inhibitory mechanisms are presumably defective in individuals with attention deficit disorder, who become so distracted by inadvertent stimuli that they have a difficult time attending to what they are supposed to be doing.[7]

Information appears to be stored in the sensory information system as a series of patterns and configurations that are networked to create representations of specific objects and events. These may be a unique record of a particular experience or a composite schema derived from a number of related experiences, such as encoding a generic representation of a dog or a chair: storing a picture of a generic dog in one's mind, together with information about how particular dogs vary from it, is more efficient than storing a picture of every dog we have ever encountered. The things with which we are most familiar, like our families, our homes, our pets, and our neighborhoods, are almost certainly stored as composite representations which can be recalled and modified to fit the memory of each particular instance in which they occur, like digital images in a computer. Much of the sensory information that is stored in the brain is probably in the form of similar representations that can be modified as needed to fit particular circumstances, rather than being separately stored every time they are experienced. This process of condensation probably occurs with most common categories of objects, so that our subsequent memories of them are to some extent reconstructed, rather than recalled exactly as originally experienced.[8]

THE SYMBOLIC INFORMATION SYSTEM

In addition to its ability to process sensory information, the human brain is uniquely programmed to process information encoded in language-related symbols. These linguistic symbols not only enable us to communicate and receive information from others, they also make it possible for us to construct a symbolic model of the universe that allows us to form abstract concepts, attribute meaning, and elucidate relationships between the entities we encounter. The symbolic system enables us to *understand* what we experience, not just record it. This liberates us in a remarkable way from the static, present-bound constraints of the sensory system we share with the other species. The symbolic models that we construct greatly enlarge our range of adaptive behavior by allowing us to anticipate and predict events, not just respond to them.

The unique capabilities of the human symbolic information system are tied closely to the evolutionary development of language. Language is the code that transforms objects into symbols that can be manipulated to form combinations not found in the world of sensory experience. A symbol is merely something that signifies something else and represents it uniquely. Verbal symbols, like the ones on this page, can be mentally arranged and rearranged without having to deal with their counterparts in the real world. However, the brain's symbolic system is based not on any language we know but on underlying lexical representations that form the basis of all of our spoken languages. Language consists of a series of integrated, neuronally encoded symbols that not only record information but also capture the spatial, temporal, and causal relationships that link events. The symbolic model we construct includes abstract representations that make it possible for us to infer meaning about the events in our lives, as well as concepts such as time, space, number, and value. Unlike the sensory system, which merely records *snapshots* of episodic events, the symbolic system's temporal dimension enables it to develop categories and generalizations, by comparing and contrasting events over time.[9]

The abstract nature of the symbols used in this system allows it to include *adjectives*, which describe objects, and *verbs*, which denote the relationships between them, neither of which exists as such in the world of ordinary sensory experience. These lexical elements enable the models we develop to greatly compress the information they contain, since they do not have to store every specific instance of every object and event we have ever experienced. The same adjectives (*big, gray, beautiful*) can be used to modify any number of noun objects (*house, cat, mountain*) without each combination having to be stored as such. Connecting verbs and adverbs, such as *grow* and *change, together* and *apart,* can likewise specify the relationship between any number of entities without having to be embedded in any particular one of them.

The most important feature of the symbolic system, however, is that it can process information independent of any external input. This enables us to create the ideas and images that characterize conscious thinking and decision making, as well as much of our non-conscious problem-solving activities. Because it is not limited by what we encounter in the real world, the symbolic system enables us to imagine and create things we have never experienced, both entities, like *unicorns, subatomic particles,* and *aliens from another planet,* and abstract concepts, like *species, bravery,* and *democracy.* The system allows us to manipulate and recombine its various symbols in a myriad of ways that nature itself is not able to accomplish.

The symbolic system processes information and evaluates its meaning by assessing how it fits with the representational model we have created. Our sensory experiences are broken down into smaller, manageable components, which are then classified, filed, stored, and integrated in a way that enables us to add them to our overall base of knowledge. Fitting the pieces of this model together is like working on a gigantic puzzle, with the gaps often being filled in with wishful thinking to give a sense of completeness. Sometimes we jump to the wrong conclusion and fill in the gaps with things that are not true, so that part of the model we construct is flawed. Sometimes our senses deceive us: we look towards the horizon and believe that the earth is flat, or see the sun rotate across the sky and think that we are at the center of the universe. We also attribute cause and effect when one event regularly follows another, even when there is no causal connection between them—such as in rainmaking ceremonies and other superstitious beliefs. We all build our own particular model of the world in this way and then interpret our subsequent experiences through its prism. The table below summarizes the major differences between the sensory and symbolic information systems.

The Sensory System	*The Symbolic System*
Processes concrete sensations as perceptual engrams	Processes abstract symbols as lexical engrams
Stores a catalog of static perceptual episodes	Creates a model with relationships and rules
Dependent on external input; limited to the present	Independent of external input; includes past and future data
Involves associations and conditioned learning	Involves knowledge, understanding, and meaning
Located primarily in occipital, temporal, and parietal cortex	Located primarily in frontal and prefrontal cortex

Our emotional responses are an integral component of our information processing apparatus. They are part of a biologically ancient system that evaluates how we *feel* about incoming sensory information. Our perceived emotions represent the informational output of this process, informing us of the potential benefits and dangers that confront us. The information that we receive from sensory receptors or that we generate in the symbolic system is essentially value-free. It does not, in itself, tell us anything about the significance of what we perceive for our own well-being or survival. The function of the emotional system is to make such value assessments, to appraise whether what we are experiencing is *good* or *bad, right* or *wrong, safe* or *dangerous, beautiful* or *ugly.*[10]

The positive/pleasurable side of each species' value system is initially comprised of things that have contributed to its reproductive success and survival during the course of evolution, while the negative/aversive side initially represents things that have been harmful to these processes. Our emotional reactions are furnished by our genes but fine-tuned by experience, differently for each species and, to some extent, for each individual. Value, like beauty, is in the eye of the beholder. Emotional appraisal is based on both evolutionary and learned utility, rather than on properties inherent in the entities themselves. For instance, rotten eggs do not smell bad because hydrogen sulfide gas has a rotten smell, nor does sugar taste sweet because "sweetness" is a property of sugar molecules. We appraise them this way because our brains have been programmed through evolution to generate pleasant sensations for those aspects of the world that potentially benefit our reproductive survival and unpleasant ones for those that are potentially detrimental to it. Since computers do not have emotions, they are not able to make such appraisals.[11]

By associating various forms of *feeling good* with what are perceived to be beneficial situations and various forms of *feeling bad* with what are perceived to be harmful ones, animals learn to adapt to what they may encounter and thereby increase their chance of survival. The initial specifications of what constitutes *good* and *bad* for each species are built into its genome, so that behaviors like feeding and reproduction that are essential for survival are neurochemically linked to positive emotions. All but the very simplest of animals are able to elaborate on these innate responses by associating them with a variety of other situations through different types of learning. The biological imperative is to maximize experiences that feel good and minimize those that feel bad—and the emotional system plays a lead role in this drama.

MAKING CONNECTIONS

The symbolic and sensory information systems are intricately interconnected, both to each other and to the emotional system. Our symbolic information-processing capabilities have been superimposed on our sensory ones during the course of evolution in ways that have co-opted their functions rather than duplicated them. When we have lunch with friends, for example, our sensory system processes the various sights, sounds, tastes, and smells that impinge on us, while our symbolic one decodes the meaning of our companions' comments and our emotional one assesses how pleasant and safe the event is. This centralized coordination of information processing ensures that the body functions as an integrated whole in its dealings with the world.

Most of our symbolic representations are linked to corresponding auditory and visual engrams in ways that enable us to animate our thoughts and dreams with sounds and pictures. The memories we recall and the scenarios we create also evoke the emotional responses associated with them through links that connect the sensory and emotional systems. We can thus move around, talk to other people, and experience what things feel like in the scenes we create in our mind. Being able to picture our thoughts and ideas this way enables us to access the emotional information associated with them, for information processed entirely in the symbolic system is devoid of such evaluative input. We can, for instance, think about the various words we could use to ask our boss for a raise or rehearse in our mind various scenarios for handling the situation, picturing how he or she would respond and experiencing how we would feel in each of them. Imagination and fantasy thus enable us to evaluate how pleasurable or otherwise a contemplated action would *feel*, producing information that adds significantly to the symbolic system's more rational analysis of the proposed action.

There is not an exact correspondence, however, between the sensory and symbolic systems. There are words like *gravity* and *electricity*, for which there are no sensory images, although we can construct visual representations of them, such as a weight for gravity or a lightning bolt for electricity. There are also sensory experiences that words are unable to describe, including most tastes, smells, and emotions, even though we try our best to find ways to characterize them. Symbolic thought that is completely abstract, as in mathematics and theoretical physics, is not connected to the emotional system, so it can be processed without being affected by personal values. The subjective pleasures created by music, visual arts, and good food, on the other hand, highlight the close connections that link the body's sensory and emotional systems. The temporal patterns invoked by music, the spatial ones by art, and the somatic ones by taste are processed initially like all other perceptual inputs, but the neuronal firing patterns they elicit are connected to allied configurations in the emotional system that generate esthetic pleasure.

NEURAL SYSTEMS

The brain is largely an information detecting, amplifying, and analyzing device. The symbolic, sensory, and emotional systems that perform these functions are layered one on top of the other in evolutionary development. Our most basic information processing apparatus is concerned with the regulation of vital biological functions, such as eating and reproduction, the next level with learning and associations, and the most advanced one with symbols and executive action. These combine to form a highly integrated system, with each adding increased functionality to the others. As MacLean (1990) has noted, this three-fold arrangement corresponds roughly to the three anatomical regions that constitute the human forebrain and reflect our evolutionary relatedness to reptiles, primitive vertebrates, and other mammals.[12]

The emotional system is one of the brain's most ancient components, being largely involved with chemical messages transmitted by the endocrine and autonomic nervous systems. It is primarily located at the center of the brain in a series of structures termed the *limbic system*. These structures, which are situated directly under the two cerebral hemispheres, have extensive neural connections to incoming sensory information and to the areas of the cortex that process it. The limbic system evaluates the potential for pleasure or pain in whatever we experience in ways that guide our behavior towards happiness and self-preservation. Addictive drugs work by artificially activating this system's pleasure-generating functions, which is why they divert their users from more productive pursuits.[13]

The sensory cortex is divided into different, modality-specific regions, each of which appraises and records a particular type of incoming information. The occipital lobe at the rear of the brain processes visual information, the temporal lobes on the side process auditory information, and the parietal lobes above them process somatic data. New imaging studies show that information from the sense organs is stored close by the cortical area in which it is initially received. The neural representations of sounds, images, and bodily sensations are organized topographically in delineated areas of the cortex, with the connections between them being activated to represent experience as a unified whole. Images are, however, not stored as facsimile pictures of people or landscapes, nor sounds as audiotapes of music or speech. Whenever we recall a given scene or event, we do not get an exact reproduction but rather a newly reconstructed version of the original. The images and sounds we conjure in our mind's eye and ear, although good replicas of what we have previously experienced, can be inaccurate or incomplete, especially in their details. Reconstituted images are also less vivid than the ones generated by stimuli from the outside.[14]

The frontal lobes of our cerebral hemispheres have undergone the greatest expansion during evolution and now encompass almost a third of our total cortical area. They are the last areas of the cortex to develop in young children and they continue to mature throughout adolescence, making them particularly susceptible to environmental influence. They are connected to every other part of the brain, and function as its overall integrator and regulator. In addition to being involved in language and symbolic modeling, they play a major role in allowing us to plan and organize our behavior. The most anterior part of this region, the prefrontal cortex, is highly developed in humans in ways that seem to facilitate our ability to handle temporal information and develop symbolic representations. The functions of the prefrontal cortex are discussed further in Chapter 15.

THE ORGANIZATION OF INFORMATION

Before we can process and store the input our senses receive, we first have to be able to perceive the *information* that it contains, to distinguish meaningful *signals* from meaningless *noise*. Information detection involves perceiving recurrent patterns in data, deviations from apparent randomness. Our brains extract information from the myriad of sensory impulses they receive by searching for underlying regularities and by analyzing the causes of variation in what we encounter, for it is only by being able to detect regularities over time that systematic variation can be perceived. A trained observer, like the fictional Sherlock Holmes, can always perceive more information than an untrained one, which is why Eskimos are apparently able to distinguish so many different types of snow.[15]

Information is contained in the way objects are arranged within a system, not in the objects themselves. If we scramble all of the letters in this paragraph, rather than having them arranged in a particular order, the information they contain is lost. No new information can be gained if all of our everyday events are experienced as separate and unrelated to each other or to the past. Growing infants slowly begin to identify repetitive patterns in the otherwise bewildering chaos that initially surrounds them. They first learn to identify that this is the same person, object, or sensation that they have experienced previously. Next they learn that some of their experiences are similar to earlier ones, and they begin to see objects as being members of a general class, such as a thing to sit on or a four-legged animal. Classification and generalizations increase the amount of organization in our internal representation systems. Repeated experiences that are recognized as being similar or associated are linked when they are stored, so that our sense of randomness and unpredictability decreases.

Information is stored in the brain as unique patterns of neuronal connectivity that encode particular deviations from randomness. These patterns do not need to have any physical resemblance to the objects or events they represent, as long as they have a unique, one-to-one correspondence with them in some other way. Just as pictures and sounds can be converted into patterns of electrical energy for television, the neural symbols that encode our experiences and ideas do not have to physically resemble them, just represent them in some unambiguous way. Neurons act as the transducers that convert information from one representational system to another by forming a pattern of connections that deviates from randomness in the same way it does in the original system. The more organized our knowledge and understanding, the less random the arrangement and activity of our cortical neurons.[16]

Meaning, relevance, and utility shape our ability to extract information from our sensory input. Several people can witness the same event and perceive virtually identical sensory data, but the information they extract from it depends in part on their past experience, their emotional response, and the personalized expectancies they bring to the situation. Despite this, we generally take our perceptions at face value, not realizing the complexity of the process that translates raw sensory input into conscious experience. When we look at a scene, what we actually experience is energy in the form of vibrations from waves of different frequencies, low frequencies for hearing and higher frequencies for vision. These electromagnetic waves interact with receptors that trigger neural codes and result in the brain's construction of a representation of the external experience. The way that each brain recreates a given scene is dependent on the information, meanings, and emotions already stored in it, and thus tends to differ from one person to the next. Most of us believe, however, that the world we see is the same one seen by others, that our perceptions of it are accurate and unbiased by our experience and beliefs—no matter the evidence to the contrary.

The final information-processing step is initiating an appropriate behavioral response, based on our evaluation of incoming data against the background of the information and beliefs we have previously acquired. Much of what we call *thinking* has to do with the abstract reasoning, envisioned try-outs, and emotional appraisals involved in these evaluations. The elaborate systems that our species has developed for processing information enable us to *decide* between alternate ways of responding to what confronts us, rather than being limited to relatively fixed ways of coping. We differ from other animals by the extent to which we can perform intentional acts based on our past experience and our personal values. Other species have only a limited ability to apply what they have learned from one situation to another. Dolphins, for instance, for all of their intelligence, are somehow unable to figure out that they could leap over the surrounding tuna nets to safety. Even chimpanzees can only discover the solution to a problem if all of the elements are readily at hand for trial and error manipulation; they cannot solve it in their mind. Reasoning and deciding are primarily about the future, about using what we have previously learned to increase our chances of achieving a distant goal.

The amount of information in a system is a measure of its degree of organization or negative entropy, since entropy represents the amount of disorganization in a system. According to the second law of thermodynamics, everything in the universe tends to increase in entropy, becoming progressively run down and disorganized over time. Biological systems are characterized, however, by their ability to counter this tendency by importing nutrient energy to help them remain in an organized state. When they are no longer able to do this, of course, they become disorganized and die. The human brain has mostly been studied as if it were a closed system without any external interactions, even though it is clearly an open one with permeable boundaries through which it is in constant interaction with its surroundings. Reductionism has been the predominant way that scientific knowledge has developed over the centuries—taking things apart to see what makes them tick, like dissecting the brain and studying its cells under the microscope. But it is not the only way. We can also understand things in terms of the systems of which they themselves are a component part. The functioning of the brain as an open system in interaction with its external environment is what we refer to as the *mind*. It can best be understood by studying how the brain as a whole processes and responds to information from its environment.[17]

CHAPTER 5

The Role of Learning and Memory

Memory is the treasury and guardian of all things.
—Marcus Cicero

Learning and memory are related aspects of the informational systems that characterize all living species. Their two functions are virtually indistinguishable at the neuronal level, because they both depend on the same changes in the synaptic connections that link nerve cells together as a result of experience. Learning allows animals to modify their subsequent behavior in response to what they experience, while memory makes it possible for them to record, store and recognize what they have previously encountered. Humans have a number of specialized capacities for *symbolic* learning and memory that are not shared by other species. These unique functions enable us to analyze our experience, build an increasingly elaborate representational model of the world, and anticipate the future.[1]

LEARNING

We are endowed with a built-in capacity to learn from what we experience, a process that evolution has molded over the millennia to broaden our range of adaptive behavior. Learning modifies our neuronal connections in such a way that we respond differently when exposed to a situation we have encountered before. There is no guarantee, of course, that what we learn is either useful or correct. There are several different types of learning, each based on a different type of neuronal processing:

- *Sensory (Conditioned) Learning.* Sensory learning involves inbuilt mechanisms that enable us to remember experiences that made us feel good, so that we can repeat them in the future, as well as ones that made us feel bad, so we can avoid them. When a mother praises her children for doing something and scolds them for doing something else, the former behavior tends to increase in frequency while the latter tends to decrease. Conditioned learning is the part of our information system that continually augments and modifies the stored repository of our sensory experiences, as well as the associations connected to them.[2]
- *Symbolic (Verbal) Learning.* Symbolic learning involves our capacity to learn from the experiences of others, as communicated through spoken and written language. We can also consciously reflect on what we experience by using internally generated words to modify how we understand the world. Verbal learning is an integral part of the symbolic information system and a major source of the data we use to make our mental models.
- *Skill Learning.* Skill learning involves learning how to perform a task that requires motor skill and coordination, such as learning how to tie our shoelaces, ride a bicycle, or play golf. It is essentially a motor learning process and is produced by the selective increase in neuronal connectivity that occurs with repeated practice at a task. Although the tasks initially require conscious effort, they become automatic once we become skilled at performing them.
- *Imitative and Identificative Learning.* Imitative and identificative learning involve learning by watching, imitating, and identifying with others. Young children are born mimics, which is how they initially learn what language to speak, what customs to follow, and what precepts to observe. They also learn much of their values, attitudes, and tastes by identifying with role models and other significant figures, including parents, teachers, athletes, and entertainers. Children can, unfortunately, also learn bigotry and intolerance through the same mechanisms. Most of the learning we acquire by imitation and identification is just "absorbed" into our belief systems without our being aware it has happened.[3]

Knowledge refers to sets of *organized information* encoded within our central nervous system. Some of it is based on our own personal experience, but most is based on the experience of others as passed on to us through culture and education. Knowledge can also be acquired through our genes, in terms of innate dispositions and tendencies based on the evolutionary experience of our species. *Understanding* is a special form of knowledge that involves knowing what causes something, what results from it, how to influence it, and how it relates to other phenomena—in other words, having a *model* of how it functions. The ultimate test of understanding is being able to predict or control whatever is being considered. The abstract thought and connections required for understanding are, however, not available in the sensory information system since they are entirely dependent on symbolic functioning.

Knowledge and understanding are related constructs that refer to the concepts, generalizations, rules, and the like that we infer from the information we have acquired. They represent the way that learned information has been integrated into our representational systems. Knowledge and understanding involve having *usable* information about a subject, such as gravity, horse racing, or tomorrow's weather. Our symbolic system organizes and compresses our experiences into increasingly abstract categories (e.g., poodle → dog → mammal → vertebrate → animal), which enable us to make generalizations and infer meaning. The more complete and organized our representational model, the more we can link ideas to understand something that is new or different. The brain's internal representation system enables us to condense the informational content of our everyday experiences by finding discernible order and regularity among them. There are, however, a number of distinct forms of knowledge, each involving a different type of symbolic linkage, such as knowing how to do something, knowing what something looks or tastes like, knowing about a property or quality of something, and knowing the feelings it engenders.[4]

Although all animals are able to learn from experience, they vary enormously in their capacity to do so. Our species is unique, however, in that we can also learn from the experiences that others convey to us through spoken and written language. Knowledge and beliefs are passed down from one generation to the next, so that we do not have to keep reinventing the wheel or rediscovering fire. Acquiring such second-hand knowledge is a hallmark of industrialized nations, and education to do so is an essential component of democratic ones. The printing press, libraries, the media, and the Internet have exponentially increased our ability to learn from the wisdom and folly that others have accumulated—although not everyone is able to take equal advantage of the opportunities these sources provide. Learning rote facts that do not fit into a pre-existing context is difficult, as every student knows. Because symbolic information is stored within hierarchically organized constructs, rather than as separate items, isolated facts are best retained by incorporating them into an appropriate representational system.[5]

MEMORY

There are at least five basic memory systems, each with its own distinct function and processing arrangement.[6]

- *Sensory (Episodic) Memory.* Sensory memory, like sensory learning, involves remembering objects and events we have previously encountered. In humans, it is primarily a visual and auditory recording system that stores the neuronal representations generated by our experience of the external world. It is comprised of discrete, time-limited episodes that can be recognized later on more readily than they can be recalled. Events that have been regularly experienced together become neuronally linked to each other, as well as to the emotional responses associated with them, so that eliciting one can prompt the memory of the other and the emotions linked to it.
- *Symbolic (Semantic) Memory.* Symbolic memory, like symbolic learning, involves remembering meanings, concepts, temporal sequences, relationships, and rules. It is closely linked to our faculty for language and to the neuronal systems that make this possible. Its memories are embedded as representations that shape our mental model of the universe.
- *Procedural Memory.* Procedural memory involves remembering how to perform a task or skill that has already been learned, such as how to sew or play the piano. It is essentially an alternative way of conceptualizing the motor system activities involved in skill learning. Procedural memory is usually spared in cases of amnesia.
- *Somatic Memory.* Somatic memory involves memory of bodily experiences, such as touch, taste, smell, and pain. Although we can

recognize new somatic experiences as being similar to previous ones, and can compare one with another, we are unable to directly recall and re-experience the tastes or smells we have previously encountered or the sensations of touch or pain we once felt.

• *Emotional Memory.* Emotional memory enables us to re-experience the emotional states associated with the events we recall. Prior emotions cannot be independently recalled, but they can be elicited by recalling or recognizing an object, event, or thought that previously evoked them. This is how many professional actors generate the emotions they portray.

RECOGNITION AND RECALL

Recognition and recall are two distinct aspects of memory. *Recognition* is the sense of familiarity elicited when a current experience activates the memory of an event previously encoded in the sensory system. *Recall,* on the other hand, is the conscious reconstruction of a previously experienced event, either cued by a current stimulus or elicited without external prompting. Recognition is associated with the sensory information system and is evident throughout the animal kingdom, while recall, particularly when un-cued, appears to be a function of the symbolic system that is limited to humans. Even with humans, however, information that is experienced as a continuous whole, such as a symphony or sunset, cannot be subsequently re-experienced, because our representational models incorporate only events that can be broken down into discrete codable elements.[7]

While we can recognize a wide variety of experiences as being similar to ones we have previously had, we are not able to recall and directly re-experience physical sensations like taste, smell, touch, or pain. We can recall that we had these "continuous" sensations and the circumstances in which we had them, but we cannot re-experience the sensations themselves in the absence of a current stimulus. Images and sounds are the primary modalities we can recall or conjure in our imagination, as well as in our dreams. We are, however, able to experience the emotions associated with the various scenarios we imagine. The hallucinatory experiences that occur in schizophrenia also involve mainly auditory and visual sensations; while olfactory and tactile hallucinations can occur, they are generally the result of direct neurological irritation or damage.[8]

Recall involves activation of information that has been processed and encoded symbolically. There are no symbolic representations of smell, taste, touch, or pain, which is why they cannot be directly recalled. In addition to their role in mediating language, the senses of vision and hearing serve biologically specialized functions that process information from distant sources, while smell, taste, touch, and pain process only information from our direct interface with the environment. These surface receptors involve an analogical form of information processing that differs from the digital type of representation our distance receptors convey in constructing a model of the outside world. Even though the symbolic memory system does not record sensory data as such, it apparently keeps track of where the *scripts* that activate particular recollections are stored—like the index of an intricately cross-referenced filing system. Different patterns of neuronal activation produce different scripts, in the form of recalled memories, imaginary scenarios, or previews of hoped-for eventualities.[9]

Our capacity for recognition is far greater than our capacity for recall. We can, for example, recognize a picture of a person we scarcely know, or the roads of a city in which we used to live, although we cannot otherwise recall them. It seems that we cannot recall experiences for which we have no discrete symbols, such as physical sensations and emotions, probably indicating that some type of symbolic representation has to be present for us to reconstruct an experience from stored sensory engrams. Familiar musical numbers can be recognized, for instance, but cannot be recalled as simulated performances, even though we may be able to hum the tunes and sing the words. There would, of course, be no need for a recording industry if we could recreate live musical performances in our minds. It also seems that we only encode enough of the properties of an object or event to be able to make the gross discriminations required in everyday life. Most of us are unable to report the markings on a dollar bill or the layout of the numbers on a telephone pad without prompting, and even experienced typists are often unable to recall the layout of the keys—although they usually can recognize the correct one when shown alternatives.[10]

Children have no recallable memory during the first few years of life—and adults cannot remember events that occurred before they were three or four years old, the time that we begin to develop a representational model of the world. Older children can, however, use play figures to act out traumatic experiences that occurred during their early years, indicating that these experiences have been recorded in their sensory memory but that they are unable to recollect them without help from prompting cues. Preschool children also have problems remembering the source of their memories, as the frontal regions responsible for this are not yet fully functional. The ability to foretell what is likely to happen in the future generally develops about the same time as the ability to recall what has happened in the past.

NEURONAL PROCESSING

Experiential memories are encoded as changed patterns of neuronal connectivity in the sensory and associational areas of the brain, while symbolic ones are apparently stored as changed neuronal linkages associated with the prefrontal cortex. These neuronal changes leave their respective imprints on us either as learned behavioral responses or increased knowledge and understanding. While our memory systems have been molded by the selective advantages they have conferred on our species over the millennia, the multitude of demands that modern societies place on them is a relatively new phenomenon. Our ancestors' minds were much less burdened with complex memories during the greater part of our evolutionary history, as they had no books, no schools, and no television—and rarely traveled to unaccustomed places or encountered unfamiliar faces.[11]

Although most of us believe that everything we learn is stored permanently in our brain, even if not always accessible, the data do not support this. We are only able to remember a small fraction of the immense number of sensory episodes we experience during a lifetime. It seems that only the essential elements of a situation are extracted and stored in memory, rather than the entire episode, so that we usually remember only the gist of an event and paint in the details from general memory sources. The only things that seem to be encoded when we record new experiences are the aspects that distinguish them from similar ones we have had in the past. Only the size, shape, and feel of a quarter need to be remembered, for instance, to identify it as a coin and discriminate it from other ones, not the information inscribed on its face. It seems that we capture the unique features of events and fill in the rest with material from generic engrams that have been previously stored. When a memory is later recalled, it is reconstituted by combining these key features with appropriate background material, much like mixing instant coffee with water. Such recalled memories can, however, be modified outside of our awareness to fit current needs and expectations, which is what makes them so troublesome when they are offered as sole testimony about some long past misdeed.[12]

We initially retain information on a temporary basis in what is termed *working memory*, which enables us to have access to it without having to incorporate it into more permanent storage. We remember a number from the phone book long enough to dial it, for instance, and then forget it. Working memory provides us with a sense of personal continuity from the recent past, through the present and into the immediate future, so that we do not experience our lives as a series of discontinuous events. Incoming information has to be encoded much more thoroughly to establish longer-term memories, a process that is facilitated by associating it with already existing knowledge. While short-term memory seems to involve an increase in the transmission of impulses over current neural pathways, long-term memory apparently requires the growth of new synaptic connections, a slower process and one that can be blocked by drugs that inhibit protein synthesis.[13]

Sensory experiences that do not reach consciousness cannot be recalled at a later date. As you read this page, for instance, the ideas are processed without the letters and words themselves entering your awareness, and these are thus not subsequently available for recall. The same process occurs with a great deal of our everyday experience, so that none of the more mundane information about our daily routines is retained. Events that enter consciousness can also get discarded, especially if held only in short-term memory, for our brains are selective about what they retain. Information about the traffic we see as we drive along the expressway does not get stored for later recall unless something unusual happens to focus our attention on it. Our sensory apparatus is not like a camera that continuously records everything we encounter, since even the prodigious storage capacity of the human brain would be overwhelmed by that amount of detail.

Forgetting is the other side of memory. We have a hard time as we get older recalling names and experiences that were not especially meaningful. Scientists who have studied this phenomenon do not know whether the brain discards memories that no longer fit into a coherent fabric or whether we have just forgotten where we placed them. Seeing a long-lost friend or a familiar photograph can prompt us to recall memories that we were not otherwise able to access, indicating that at least some of this information is still there. We lose some of our overall brain mass every decade as we age, with the frontal areas being most affected. Elderly individuals tend to forget the sources of particular memories, cannot always remember the temporal sequences of events, and perform significantly worse in tests of recall than on ones of recognition. It makes sense from a biological point of view to believe that the synaptic connections that link the brain's neurons weaken over time if they are not used, just as those that are used frequently become stronger. Thankfully, we do not need to remember everything that has ever happened to us.[14]

FORETELLING THE FUTURE

The recall of past experiences can be activated through both voluntary and involuntary mechanisms. *Associative retrieval* is an involuntary process of recall elicited by experiencing an event that is similar to a previously experienced one or by language associated with it. *Strategic retrieval*, on the other hand, is a voluntary recall process accomplished through consciously searching one's memory stores for a particular recollection, somewhat like finding a book in a library. The verbal stimuli that prompt it can be generated either by external cues or by one's own internal thoughts and fantasies. Strategic retrieval is the search and recall process that gets initiated when an examination question reads, for instance, "What were the three main causes of the fall of the Roman Empire?" or a detective asks, "Where were you between eight and ten o'clock on the night of January 8th?" It is an *intentional* process that only humans seem to possess.[15]

Strategic retrieval is usually initiated through language that reactivates the engrams that contain the particular memory. We apparently employ the same process to generate the imaginary scenarios we use to think and plan about the future; that is, we generate thoughts and images about the future by using the same mechanisms we use to recall the past. Just as *re-calling* the past involves re-constructing what happened from stored events in our representational models, *fore-telling* the future involves creating imaginary scenarios from the same components. The symbolic information system enables us to call-up both past events and future scenarios at will, without having to be prompted by what is going on in our current environment. Recalling the past and foretelling the future both depend on the representational models we have constructed and the integrity of our prefrontal cortex. This area of the brain organizes incoming information by creating a time and source tag for the engrams our sensory system generates. These tags play a critical role in strategic thinking by allowing us to remember where and when previous events took place and to forecast where and when future ones will likely happen. Individuals with impaired prefrontal function cannot recall the past or foretell the future in a meaningful way.[16]

Prospective memory involves recalling things that have not yet happened, such as what we plan to do, and how, when, and where we thought about doing it. Most people in technologically advanced societies spend a considerable amount of their time recalling plans and ideas about the future, such as where and when they are supposed to meet a friend or what they intend to do or say about a particular matter. Planning involves a kind of problem solving by mental simulation—envisioning the prospective circumstances, mentally running through a number of possible scenarios, and selecting the one with the most promising prospects. We remember these ideas and expectations about the future in the same way that we remember our experiences of the past.[17]

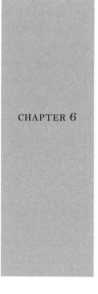

CHAPTER 6

The Impact of Consciousness

> *Freedom stretches only as far as the*
> *limits of consciousness.*
> —Carl Jung

The word *consciousness* is used to refer to two distinct but related phenomena, one of which is a function of the sensory information system and the other a function of the symbolic one. The first simply involves an awareness of the sensory stimuli that are currently being perceived by an individual. We use this meaning when we say that someone is conscious in the sense of not being *unconscious*, or that someone has regained *consciousness*. The second use refers to a subjective experience of being able to sense our own existence, to choose what we do, to recall events from the past, and to think about the future—and be aware that we are doing these things. It is a distinctly human experience that rests on our ability to process symbolic information and develop representational models of our world. Consciousness provides the infrastructure that enables us to experience time and develop a sense of the past and the future.[1]

DEFINITION

Some of the confusion in trying to understand the nature of consciousness has to do with the various ways its sensory and symbolic aspects are defined. They are differentiated here by using the term *consciousness* to refer exclusively to the self-awareness type of experience that occurs in humans, and the term *sentience* to denote the sensory abilities that we share with other species. Several writers fail to make this distinction; these include Baars (1997), Crick (1994), and Humphrey (1992). But most do, although without a consensus about how to name these two different states. Edelman (1992), for instance, refers to them as *primary consciousness* and *higher order consciousness*, while Mandler (1997) calls them *consciousness* and *reflective consciousness*, and Damasio (1999) *consciousness* and *extended consciousness*. Whether we believe that consciousness is limited to humans, present in other primates, or widespread throughout the animal kingdom largely depends on how we define it.[2]

Consciousness, at least as here defined, refers to a complex phenomenon comprising at least six distinct components, usually experienced one at a time. These different types of subjective experience, which describe consciousness as much as they define it, are as follows:

- *Sensory Awareness.* An appreciation of environmental and somatic information currently being registered by our sensory receptors.
- *Thinking.* A process of self-dialogue which uses words generated by our symbolic information system to solve problems, make decisions, reflect on environmental happenings, and rehearse anticipated conversations.
- *Memory and Imagination.* A process of mentally experiencing auditory and visual scenes generated by our sensory and symbolic information systems, including recollections of past events, anticipations of future ones, and imaginary scenarios.
- *Self-awareness.* A subjective awareness of our own existence as an individual distinct from others, as either an initiator or a recipient of action. This includes our senses of free will and personal identity.
- *Emotional Awareness.* An awareness of our current mood and feelings, which is usually experienced as an accompaniment to one of the above components and reflects the emotional state associated with it.
- *Time Awareness.* A general awareness of the passage of time that is based on our ability to recall the past and anticipate the future. This is disrupted by events and substances that focus our attention on the present.

SENTIENCE

Sentience refers to the appreciation of current sensory and somatic stimuli. It is somewhat like the experience we have when we are intensely focused in the present, completely absorbed in a current task, or lost in daydreams or a trance. During such times there is little subjective sense of consciousness, since there is a virtual absence of self-awareness, spontaneous thought, or the sense of time. We are only dimly aware of what else is going on around us, and experiences are dealt with on a semi-automatic basis. Sentient awareness is how young children and nonhuman primates appear to experience the world, as well as the way our far-distant ancestors presumably did. Consciousness is not essential for responding to sensory perceptions, or even for learning from them, but it is required for having them incorporated into the fabric that makes up our representational model of the world.

Sentient awareness is necessary, but not sufficient, for the experience of consciousness, as it does not include our experience of ourselves as autonomous, decision-making beings. As Damasio (1999) notes, *sentience* "provides the organism with a sense of self about one moment—now—and about one place—here. . . . it does not illuminate the future, and the only past it vaguely lets us glimpse is that which occurred in the instant just before. There is no elsewhere, there is no before, there is no after." *Consciousness*, he maintains, "provides the organism with an elaborate sense of self—an identity and a person, you or me, no less—and places that person at a point in individual historical time, richly aware of the lived past and of the anticipated future."

The special type of consciousness that we possess has undoubtedly evolved from primitive types of sentience, just as the unique features of our brain have evolved from more rudimentary ones. The evolutionary continuum that determines the degree to which a species' nervous system has a central, brainlike structure determines how its sensory experiences are perceived and integrated. All species are not equally sentient, nor sentient in the same way; those that are most closely related to us probably are most like us in their sentient experiences. Self-awareness, free will, and the sense of time are, however, exclusively human experiences. Consciousness can expose humans to pleasures and anxieties that other sentient creatures never know. No other animal appears to be able to re-experience past events, contemplate self-generated ideas, or predict the longer-term outcome of their behavior. Griffin (1976) quotes Whitehead: "The distinction between men and animals is in one sense only a difference in degree. But the extent of the degree makes all the difference."[3]

It is not profitable to get into a debate about whether other animals are endowed with consciousness or whether they possess the sort of thoughts and feelings we do. As already mentioned, it all depends on how these are defined. The experience of human consciousness, however, involves having access to our unique information processing systems; "animal consciousness," whatever it is, is not the same thing. As far as we can tell, other animals do not possess the neuronal capability for constructing a symbolic model of the universe—and are thus limited to processing present-oriented experiences. Although they obviously can learn from what they experience and exhibit evidence of memory and intelligence, we stand alone in our ability to transcend time and respond to anticipated eventualities that are independent of our present circumstances. Kinget (1987) observes, "Animals exist physically, but not experientially, in that mysterious time-space we call the world. They have no sense of time except for some awareness of the immediate before and after, for their world is bound by the senses, and time is not a sensory datum. This places the non-human animal outside the universe of symbols (though not of signs) and consequently outside the universe of time."

There undoubtedly is a fundamental continuity between mankind and the other species, including a high likelihood that a number of them have developed simple forms of symbolic representation. Chimpanzees and dolphins show considerable evidence of intelligence and possess sophisticated communication skills, but these do not necessarily signify that they have a human type of consciousness. Although dogs and other social species appear to consider alternate modes of action, anticipate short-term consequences, experience a range of emotional expression, and recognize individual members of their own kind, it does not necessarily mean that they have a symbolic representation *system*. They may experience loss, the pain of separation, and difficulty in abandoning a dead companion, but presumably without connection to their own potential mortality—and without the type of self-awareness that characterizes human consciousness.

Most other animals experience some sort of sentient awareness as it pertains to the present but not to the past and future. They can recognize entities they have previously encountered, but they cannot otherwise recall them. They can respond to sensory cues in complex ways, based on both learning and genetic programming, but they cannot initiate action independent of them. Their form of consciousness is time-bound and sensory in nature, like that of human infants. The capabilities that our symbolic representation system confers on us represent a distinction that cannot be minimized. In fact, it is precisely because of *our* special abilities that we have a moral responsibility to treat other species with respect and to protect them from unnecessary suffering. Mammals and other higher vertebrates are clearly sentient creatures that feel pain and distress, and they should be treated humanely because *we* are moral beings, not because they are. That we do not expect them to show the same kind of consideration to other species highlights the fact that we do not believe they are capable of the conscious self-determination this requires. The enormity of the consciousness gap between us and even our nearest relatives in no way denigrates them; it just underscores our unique place in nature's grand design.

The topic of animal consciousness is a highly controversial one that is frequently colored by beliefs that other species have rights similar to ours—although not similar responsibilities. As we will likely never know what any other species actually *experiences*, it is a question that can be settled only through indirect evidence. Those who argue that other species have consciousness generally treat other animals as a unitary group, not recognizing the differences in brain structure and complexity among them. If, for instance, we do not draw a line between apes and humans with regard to consciousness, is there anywhere else where it should be drawn between mammals, invertebrates, insects, and protozoa? It seems best to separate the scientific questions about animal consciousness from the moral ones about how we should treat other species. Walker (1983) believes it makes sense to suppose that awareness and mental organization occur in animals, but he cautions whether nonverbal animals actually have consciousness. He quotes Schopenhauer (1788–1860): "Animals live in the present and are incapable of reflecting on past and future events (in particular their own death), and cannot form abstract conceptions."[+]

CONSCIOUS EXPERIENCE

Consciousness is the private arena in which we live our lives. It is an elusive and poorly understood phenomenon, one of those ineffable things that everyone knows but no one can quite describe. The experience of consciousness involves more than a simple awareness of what is going on, for it also includes a sense of having an observing *self* that monitors and directs what is being experienced. As well as being aware of the flowers we see in the vase, we are also aware that we are seeing them—and know that we can shift our attention elsewhere if we wish. Our experience of consciousness would not be the same if we were only able to be passively aware of everything, without having any sense of our own capacity to influence the content of our subjective world. In fact, we would probably not *experience* it at all if we were merely spectators to life's events. Tye (1995) believes that consciousness is the central mystery of human experience and probably the ultimate scientific frontier, something that has baffled philosophers down through the ages, and still does.

Consciousness has been likened to a *theater of the mind*, a venue in which issues that are of pertinence to us get played out for us to experience and consider. It is really more like an interactive television of the mind which we control by switching between channels and choosing the content of the dramas being shown. We can choose to view live programming, by zooming in and out of our current environment, or archival reruns of previous dramas in which we participated, or simulated scenes of anticipated events and make-believe scenarios. Most of these programs go on whether we watch them or not, just like the ones on television, for the brain keeps on processing the information they contain outside of our awareness. Consciousness is notoriously difficult to study, however, not just because of its inaccessibility to objective scrutiny, but also because of its elusive subjectivity, since once we start thinking about what we are thinking, we are no longer thinking it.[5]

The experiences that characterize human consciousness are a function of the unique ways we process information. Our ability to imagine and think about events that are not related to our current sensory input would not be possible if we did not have a symbolic representational system with which to generate them. This system's models enable us to live in two parallel worlds, a public one that we share with everyone else and a private one that is largely of our own making. Consciousness is what makes it possible for us to sense our private universe, be aware of its time scales, and switch between it and the public one at will. This ability to choose what we are aware of and shift from the world of sensory perceptions to the world of mental representations is what makes the *experience* of consciousness possible. Creatures that are time-bound to the present, whatever their sense and awareness of the world, do not have the same subjective experience.

Consciousness is experienced in real time, one item after the other in orderly sequence. Most of the brain does not function this way, since it operates primarily as a parallel processing system that deals with items simultaneously, rather than sequentially. Greenfield (1995) has suggested that the biological function of consciousness is to act as a kind of gatekeeper that makes sure that only one of the multiple sources of information being processed gets acted upon at a time. Consciousness thus helps transform the brain's parallel processing operation into a sequential one that allows language to be transmitted and received in a comprehensible order, one word following after the other in a clearly evident sequence. Whatever way the brain encodes the neurochemical symbols that represent language, the sequential processing ability of consciousness is the link that enables us to translate these into meaningful discourse. Consciousness is probably as necessary for the experience of language as language is for the experience of consciousness.[6]

Consciousness serves multiple purposes. Information that is processed outside of consciousness cannot be recalled later on, so that animals that lack a human-type consciousness are not able to recollect what happened in the past or plan what they hope to achieve in the future. Their central nervous systems can be modified by experience without their ever being aware of it, just as their immune systems can, and they can recognize objects and events as similar to past ones, but they cannot spontaneously recall or re-experience them. Consciousness is necessary for the accumulation of abstract knowledge and understanding that characterizes our species, as well as for the ability to make moral choices. Thinking is like speaking to oneself, a conscious and language-related process that has to be performed serially in order to be intelligible. Often we do not know what we really think until we put our thought into words, as one of E. M. Forster's characters observes: "How do I know what I think until I see what I say?"[7]

HOW IS THE CONTENT DETERMINED?

All of us have a sense of being able to choose what we consciously pay attention to, which part of the environment we focus on, which memory we recall, which fantasy we imagine, or which problem we consider. Our sense that there is a little *me* located somewhere inside our head making these decisions is part of our experience of our self as an agent and initiator, rather than a passive responder, part of our sense of possessing free will. But there is no little person in there at the controls, just a number of scattered neurons organized in some far from understood pattern—a decision-making process, but no *decider.*

All of us also have had the experience of something intruding on its own into our consciousness, independent of our choosing. The body clearly has a set of informational priorities, any one of which can preempt whatever else is currently occupying our attention. These include alarms that indicate the presence of external danger, internal signals of distress like pain and hunger, and states of emotional and sexual arousal. Certain stimuli grab our attention, like the smell of something burning, a creak on the stairs at night, the sound of someone in distress, or a sudden change in our surroundings. Creative thinking and future planning can only take place when we are not occupied with more pressing matters.[8]

We normally focus most of our attention on the matter at hand, be this work, social interaction, or entertainment. The lights are dimmed when we go to the theater or the movies so that we can focus on the show without being distracted. We can get so lost in a good performance that we forget for a while whatever else is on our mind. Soldiers in the midst of battle and football players during an exciting game can be so engrossed in what is going on that they do not feel pain when they are injured. Fears and worries, on the other hand, distract us from giving our full attention to what we are doing—which can be dangerous if we are flying a plane or performing surgery. We can, however, attend to more than one task at a time thanks to our dual information processing systems. Experienced motorists can focus their attention on planning a future activity as they drive along the expressway, although inexperienced ones still need to devote their attention to driving if they are to do so safely.

Some people focus their attention so exclusively on one or other aspect of consciousness that it interferes with their overall level of mental well-being. Obsessive worriers are so involved in introspection that they have little awareness of their current environment or own emotional state, a condition referred to as *isolation of affect*. Hypochondriacs focus their consciousness excessively on their visceral sensations, while paranoid individuals focus theirs on the external environment. The conscious experience of depressed individuals is full of unbidden thoughts of doom, while that of anxious ones is awash with specters of disaster. It seems that many troubled individuals have difficulty regulating the content of their consciousness. Mental well-being involves maintaining an equilibrium among our different modes of conscious experience in order to keep thinking, feeling, and behaving in a functional balance.

THOUGHTS AND FEELINGS

Our conscious thoughts are like a form of interior dialogue that depends on the use of words and other symbols. Thinking involves the transformation of neural symbols into the kind of sequential structure that spoken language requires. We are not able to think about something consciously if we do not have a word or other symbol for it, just as we are not able to talk about something if we do not have language to describe it. We can nonetheless picture things in our minds for which we have no words, such as a friend's face, a work of art, or the scene of a disaster. Abstract concepts and ideas can also be associated with images that are brought to mind as we think about them. These are generally composite schemas, like the generic pictures that we conjure up to make a *"motion picture"* in our mind of what is happening as we read a novel, hear a story, or develop a mental scenario.

Intellect, imagination, and emotion are the major tools of consciousness. Intellect is composed of logical operations that involve the manipulation of words and other symbols to form various information-containing propositions. Intellect, by itself, contains no imagery or emotion. Imagination, on the other hand, involves conjuring up stored visual and auditory images, and stringing them together into scenarios that can be played out in our *theater of the mind.* We are not conscious of the actual scripts we have constructed as we picture these stories and experience the emotions associated with them, just as we are unaware of the actual words we see when we read a novel. Pleasant and unpleasant emotions are experienced in response to input from our self-generated ideas and images, much as they are from our sensory input. Abstract thought and reasoning do not generate emotions by themselves, although they can elicit images that make this information available.

FANTASY AND IMAGINATION

Fantasy and imagination allow us to experience life vicariously and experiment by trying things out in our mind's eye. We can use them to foresee the likely outcomes of our actions or to create make-believe worlds of our own choosing. The advantage that imagination has over pure thought is that it can elicit associated emotional information that can be used in decision making. We can thus evaluate alternative scenarios in our mind by experiencing whether they elicit favorable or unfavorable emotional reactions. Initiating future-oriented behavior depends on being able to conjure up mental scenarios that generate hopeful feelings about achieving a desired goal. What each of us is capable of imagining is limited, however, by our particular experience and understanding. We can only imagine the future in ways that are related to how we have experienced and understood the past, for we are unable to conceive of things that do not fit with our preconceived models of the world. Because of this, most people believe that angels have wings and halos and that extraterrestrial aliens come with egg-shaped heads and saucer-shaped vehicles.

Although our fantasies can contain images of things that we have never actually seen, they are created from components with which we are already familiar. Our dreams and nightmares are fashioned out of elements we already know, in much the same way that fairy tales are limited by what seems plausible to young children and science fiction by extensions of what is already known. Even the delusions of psychotic individuals are limited by how they understand the world. Individuals who used to believe they were being influenced by a radio transmitter that had been inserted in their brain now believe a computer chip is the culprit. Every great invention and discovery was created by the combining of existing elements in some unique way in someone's mind. Ideas and images concocted out of the figments of imagination have, however, motivated people to cross oceans, build pyramids, and create civilizations. The richness of our imagination depends on the richness of our storehouse of data and the ingenuity with which we combine its elements. People who are unusually good at creating imaginary scenarios write novels and dramas to entertain and enrich those not so gifted.

FREE WILL

Consciousness is what enables us to have a choice in what we respond to and how we respond to it. We can use the model of the world we have constructed to consider various behavioral options and anticipate their future outcomes before deciding which one to pursue. We can choose from a number of present-oriented actions to help meet our currents needs or from a variety of future-oriented ones aimed at enhancing our subsequent well-being. We can also choose to focus so exclusively on the present that we forget our troubles for a while, or to disengage and indulge in reverie and fantasy. We are thus no longer captives of our circumstances, and our fate is no longer completely at the mercy of whatever happens to befall us. Our sense of free will depends on the fact that the future is not completely predictable. We have the option of choosing between actions that will lead to outcomes that we perceive as having some likelihood of taking place and of being of value to us. Our sense of choice is dependent on which of these alternative paths we decide to follow, since we would have little choice about how we responded if we already knew what would actually happen. Churchland (1996) believes that choosing where to focus what he calls our *steerable attention* may be the closest we get to freely determining our behavior.

Only as a sense of conscious choice develops is there any meaning to morality, to right and wrong, good and evil. We have no personal responsibility for what we do if our behavior is determined by forces beyond our control. A sense of the future is required for morality to develop beyond a set of rudimentary taboos, for it is the *consequences* of our actions that ultimately determine whether they are morally good or bad. Under the law, guilt is determined by what individuals *intended* to be the outcome of their actions, not just the actions themselves. Free will involves being able to choose what we pay attention to, what we make of it, and how we respond to these perceptions. Young children and severely retarded, disturbed, or demented individuals, do not share our sense of free will, because they have only a limited capacity for making such choices. This is also true of other species.[9]

Free will depends on being conscious of oneself as an independent entity in space and time, a thinker who can choose what to consider, an actor who can choose what to watch and what to do. Such self-awareness also involves an appreciation that we have a unique personal history that will one day come to an end because we are mortal. Consciousness thus comes with a price. We have to accept responsibility for our actions because of it, as well as wrestle with concerns about our own mortality and the meaning of life. It is probably no coincidence that the world's great religions emerged at about the same time that mankind seems to have acquired a fully human type of consciousness. The story of Adam and Eve in the Garden of Eden can be seen as a mythical portrayal of this transition, in which eating the fruit of the tree of knowledge symbolizes becoming conscious and bringing to an end a world of innocence and bliss. While gaining consciousness made Adam and Eve aware of themselves and of their potential for good and evil, it left them burdened with having to take responsibility for their actions, as these were now matters of choice rather than necessity.[10]

Our sense of free will is, in some ways, partly an illusion. Our behavior is mostly determined by built-in optimizing rules and strategies that analyze the potential outcomes of the various choices that confront us. It may *look* as if it is purposive by seeming to be designed to achieve some end, just like natural selection looks like it is purposive. Making oneself do something that one does not feel like doing, like getting out of bed on a cold morning, certainly feels like a willed action, even if the decision is really made by a series of interacting neurons, rather than by a *me*. Philosophers argue that we cannot be responsible for our actions if our behavior is really determined by what is encoded in our neuronal systems, if our sense of free will is nothing more than an artificial by-product of consciousness. Being *held responsible* under the law is, however, a social construct, not a scientific one. A society can establish consequences to punish deviant and unacceptable behavior—and its members need to incorporate this knowledge into their world view and be mindful of it as they choose what to do. Holding people responsible for knowingly breaking societal rules does not have to depend on whether they really have free will.

THE UNCONSCIOUS

The word *unconscious* can refer to a state of diminished arousal and awareness (as when someone is asleep or in a coma), a process of perceiving and thinking that takes place outside of our awareness (non-conscious mental activity), or a place where potentially harmful information is kept out of our awareness (*the* unconscious of Freud). Non-conscious, automatic information processing probably represents the greater part of our mental activity. It goes on day in and day out while we are awake and when we are asleep, checking incoming stimuli, solving problems that have been on our mind, and reorganizing our representational models of the universe. The fact that information processing goes on outside of awareness is evident when the solution to a problem we have been worrying about suddenly pops into our consciousness, or when we are jolted out of our sleep by the presence of a strange noise or odor. Learning can also take place outside of awareness, as with conditioning and identification, but recallable memories are not generated unless an event is first experienced consciously. Information that is processed outside of awareness can, at times, be made accessible to consciousness. When we sit down to write, for instance, we make ourselves think of the idea we wish to express, but we do not have to think of all the words—they just come into consciousness from somewhere. We are also not usually conscious of choosing the exact words we are going to use when we speak, just the point we want to make.

We are usually unaware of a great deal of the information accumulated in the representational models we have constructed, including some of our fundamental ideas and values. Our unconscious thoughts and desires may, as a result, be in conflict at times with our professed beliefs, leaving us confused about what to do. We may even find ourselves motivated by unconscious urges to behave in ways that are at odds with our avowed beliefs, as in the case of compulsive gambling or shoplifting. We may also have experienced traumatic events which we are now unaware of, especially if they occurred when we were young. Freud thought that this inaccessible information was actively repressed in some way in order to keep its upsetting content hidden from us. One of the reasons we are unable to recall early experiences may simply be that they happened before we had a fully developed consciousness and thus could not integrate them into our mental models. Repression is, however, just one of a number of the mental defense mechanisms that keep upsetting information out of conscious awareness, with denial, displacement, and rationalization being others. All of them involve a short-circuiting of our regular information processing mechanisms in order to protect us from being overwhelmed by unpleasant or unacceptable realities. They can serve a highly adaptive function, especially in the short-run.[11]

ALTERED STATES

The altered states of consciousness brought about by various mind-altering drugs or by meditative practices appear to take place by diminishing consciousness, rather than by expanding it. The heightened sensory awareness that characterizes these altered states obliterates other sources of conscious experience, enabling the individual to enter into an entirely sentient condition. Focusing intensely on here-and-now input from the sensory system results in a loss of the senses of time and self-awareness that characterize true consciousness. These states are thus experienced as a retreat from the burdens of worry and responsibility that consciousness ordinarily entails, although they also bring with them a concomitant decrease in active coping ability.

With practice and self-discipline, people who subscribe to the more meditative religions can lose all awareness of their own being and experience a transcendental sense of oceanic fusion with the universe. This is the basis of mystical trances—and, to a lesser extent, of the sense of release associated with activities like sailing, listening to music, and jogging. The more people focus their conscious awareness on a present task, the less they are aware of their troubles and concerns, which is why such activities can be experienced as pleasantly relaxing. Age-old ways of fighting bodily needs involve loosening the mind's attachment to consciousness through activities that involve intense concentration on the present, such as fasting, chanting, dancing, spinning, gazing at a mandala, or endlessly repeating a given phrase. As Alcoholics Anonymous recognizes in its advice to live one day at a time, most of what troubles us resides in our concerns about the past and our apprehensions about the future.[12]

Enhanced sentience also seems involved in the state of "flow" that Csikszentmihalyi (1990) popularized as an optimal experience that can enable people to achieve a richer, more fulfilling, more joyous sense of being alive. He described "flow" as a state in which one becomes so immersed in the present moment that "there is no room in your awareness for conflicts or contradictions; it is so perfect you want to immerse yourself completely in the experience. A person in *flow* is completely focused. There is no space in consciousness for distracting thoughts, irrelevant feelings. Self-consciousness disappears, yet one feels stronger than usual. The sense of time is distorted: hours seem to pass by in minutes." Csikszentmihalyi (1997) postulated that "flow" involves activities that are rewarding in and of themselves, rather than being aimed at achieving some later pleasure, and represents a pure experience of the present, untrammeled by worries about the past or the future. He characterizes it as a "holistic sensation that people feel when they act with total involvement. It involves a merging of action and awareness. The person is aware of his actions, but not of the awareness itself." This lack of awareness of oneself as a separate entity leads to the sense of fusion with the world that occurs during such experiences.[13]

Under conditions of extreme sensory deprivation, the only available option for consciousness is to focus on internally generated stimuli—which is why people begin to hallucinate when the deprivation is prolonged. The thought control exercised by various cults involves taking charge of an individual's consciousness by bombarding it with carefully selected sensory data and depriving it of other types of information. Hypnosis is another way of exclusively focusing an individual's attention, so that the hypnotist's instructions become the only information available for conscious processing. The mind-altering drugs that distort conscious experience also appear to do so by heightening external perception, stimulating mood states, or generating unusually vivid imagery. As Greenfield (2000) notes, the consumption of alcohol and marihuana bring about "a disconnection with the ordinary world of worries and expectations," and produce "a drift away from abstracted logical reasoning tendencies that characterize the human mind in favor of a more emotional perspective, one focused on the immediate here and now, the very features that characterize the perspective of the small child."

CHAPTER 7

Emotion as Information

> *Man ought to know that from nothing else but the brain come joys, delights, laughter, sorrows, griefs and lamentation.*
>
> —Hippocrates

Emotions are part of a relatively primitive information system that we share in some form or other with the rest of the animal kingdom. All living creatures have a built-in genetic imperative to behave in ways that maximize certain experiences and minimize others in order to promote their survival and that of their species. Things that help them achieve this, like food and sex, are thus linked with agreeable emotions and ones that threaten to harm them with disagreeable ones. Every species differs, however, in what makes it feel good and what makes it feel bad, for each has its own specific life-sustaining agenda. As Damasio (1999) notes: "Emotions are part and parcel of the regulation we call homeostasis. They are part of the machinery with which organisms regulate survival."[1]

FEELING GOOD, FEELING BAD

Emotions are one of the main sources of the subjective *feelings* that color and give meaning to our daily lives. Along with our physical senses of taste, smell, and touch, and our somatic ones of pain, distress, and discomfort, they make up the bulk of the subjective sensations that characterize our experience of consciousness. These different types of *feelings* all function as part of a biologically ancient feedback network that sustains life by maintaining a homeostatic balance, both within the organism and between it and the external environment. In the same way that sensory receptors convey information about objects and events in our environment and somatic ones tell us how our bodies are currently functioning, emotions provide information about the nature of our *relationship* with the world in which we live. They function as part of a regulatory loop that elicits the physiological and behavioral responses that help us adapt to changes in our sensory input. Despite their apparent diversity, all of these various feeling states fall into one of two broad groupings: agreeable sensations, which signify that things are all right, and disagreeable ones, which signal that something is wrong. Bentham (1789) observed that "nature has placed mankind under the governance of two sovereign masters, *pain* and *pleasure*. It is for them alone to point out what we ought to do, as well as to determine what we shall do."[2]

Our emotions convey information about changes in our relationship with the external environment. Pleasant ones (*feeling good*) indicate that all is well with the world, while unpleasant ones (*feeling bad*) signal that something is amiss—and mobilize us to change our behavior to deal with it. The behavioral responses associated with feeling bad are aimed at restoring a sense of well-being, while those associated with feeling good endeavor to maintain the current state of affairs. Emotional information thus helps us steer a safe passage in our day-to-day lives by adapting our behavior to the demands of our physical and social environments. Johnston (1999) conceptualizes our emotional system as "a kind of gyroscope that tries to guide us safely through our daily activities." As Figure 2 illustrates, the basic strategy is relatively simple—pleasurable emotions indicate a need to maintain or increase current behavior, while distressing ones indicate a need to decrease or change it.[3]

THE VARIETIES OF EMOTIONAL EXPERIENCE

Everyone knows what emotion is until they are asked to define it. One reason for this is that the term is a convenient label for a wide variety of subjective experiences, each of which has evolved for a different adaptive purpose. Some emotions, such as those associated with reproduction and feeding, serve fundamental biological needs, while others provide information about the prospect of achieving acquired goals and expectations. Some are associated with distinctive physiological responses, some with characteristic patterns of nonverbal expression, and some with extensive cognitive appraisal, but few share all these features. This is why there is no

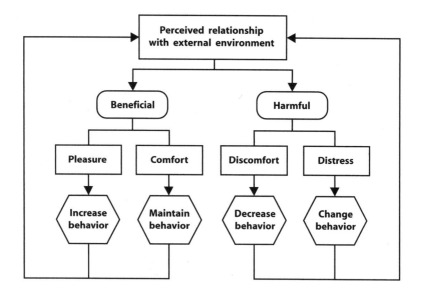

Figure 2. Emotional Information in the Regulation of Behavior

generally agreed-upon way of categorizing the emotions. Experts are not sure, for instance, whether boredom and excitement are moods or emotions, loneliness and curiosity are emotions or ideas, and optimism and greed are emotions or personality traits. The following classification is presented simply as a way of illustrating the types of information that emotions convey about our relationship with our surroundings:[4]

- *Current-state Emotions.* These convey information about the overall state of our current relationship with the world around us; they include happiness, unhappiness, pleasure, sadness, dissatisfaction, contentment, enjoyment, and delight.
- *Affiliative Emotions.* These convey information about the desirability or undesirability of engaging another person or object; they include love, hate, like, dislike, disapproval, jealousy, envy, pity, contempt, lust, loathing, resentment, despising, detesting, disgust, scorn, and revulsion. Affiliative emotions lead us either to seek other entities or to withdraw from them.[5]
- *Defensive Emotions.* These convey information about potential danger; they include concern, worry, anxiety, apprehension, fear, alarm, terror, and dread. Threatening stimuli are able to elicit rapid vis-

ceral and behavioral responses without having to wait for conscious appraisal.

- *Hostility Emotions.* These convey the information that our body, territory, property, beliefs, or expectations are being harmed or violated, or are in danger thereof; they include irritation, annoyance, frustration, anger, and rage.

- *Prospective Emotions.* These convey information about our anticipated future relationship with the external world; they include excitement, anxiety, elation, hope, desire, despair, and depression. They are the product of imagined scenarios rather than direct sensory experience.

- *Retrospective Emotions.* These convey information about our past interactions with the world; they include guilt, regret, and remorse. Both retrospective and prospective emotions are discussed further below.

- *Moral Emotions.* These convey information about our conformity with socially derived standards of what is right and wrong; they include pride, guilt, embarrassment, humiliation, and shame.

- *Esthetic Emotions.* These convey information about the beauty inherent in nature, religious experience, and certain man-made objects; they include feelings of harmony, peace, wonder, and awe.

One of the difficulties in trying to classify emotions is that the verbal labels we use to describe them fail to capture the complex subjective experiences they involve. Some emotions, such as anxiety and guilt, are thus included in more than one of the above categories, while others, like indignation and gratitude, do not fit any of them. Because our emotions are private, nonconsensual experiences, we have no way of knowing how anyone else *feels* during a given emotional experience other than through the labels they use to tell us about it. Describing emotions is like describing colors, for our visual experiences of hue are processed through similar mechanisms. This may be why we describe some emotions with terms like feeling *blue* or seeing *red*, and mix different feeling states together to create new shades and complexions.[6]

EMOTIONS AS INFORMATION

The function of the emotional system is to evaluate the adaptive importance of in-coming sensory data by determining whether our perceptions feel good or feel bad in comparison to some type of internal yardstick. It accomplishes this by comparing the pattern of the incoming sensory stimuli against innate or learned patterns of neuronal connectivity, with the various emotions representing the output of these evaluations. In humans, this process appraises both *on-line* (here-and-now) sensory stimuli and *off-line* (past and future) scenarios generated by internal representations. The raw data received by our sensory receptors are value-free, for they do not contain any information about the meaning or significance of what is being perceived. As Johnston (1999) points out, "the environment is filled with lawful and consistent events, but such happenings are devoid of all meaning, for the laws of physics and chemistry that govern the behavior of these events have no inherent purpose or intention." Value assessment is the job of the emotional system, which alerts us to whether what we are experiencing is likely to help or hinder our well-being or survival and prompts us to respond accordingly.[7]

The various kinds of feelings we experience represent the output of an appraisal process that provides information about the *relationship* between the individual and external objects and events rather than about the objects and events themselves. This process compares what is being experienced against an internal yardstick in order to assess how well the one matches the other. The informational output of these comparisons is *analogical* in nature, and this is part of what makes emotions and the other feeling states difficult to describe. Feelings can only tell us how well something matches a given standard, whether it is a good or a bad fit, but not how or why this is so. Dehaene (1997) notes that an entity is said to operate *analogically* when it performs computations by manipulating *continuous* physical quantities which are *analogous* to the variables being represented.

Analogical outputs are similar to the type of information we get when we put our hand in a tub of water—we can tell whether it is hot or cold but not what the temperature is. While our own body temperature serves as the basis for comparison in this example, we have no idea about the nature of the reference standards involved in the generation of emotional information. Some of these are obviously built-in genetically, like the sense of pleasure associated with food and sex, the sense of fear associated with threats of bodily harm, and the aversion associated with bad tastes or odors. Other comparison standards are learned from experience and from family and societal values, like the feeling of shame when we fail to live up to internalized ideals or the sense of guilt when we transgress moral expectations.[8]

Emotions and the other feeling states convey a primitive, preverbal type of information. Unlike the quantitative, digital-type information that words and numbers provide, the informational content of feeling states is qualitative and continuous in nature—and thus cannot be combined and recombined to produce generalizations or work out how things fit together. Analogical information is not amenable to the same kind of cognitive processes that make human thought and rationality possible, for it is inherently limited to matching one pattern against another to see how they compare: like or unlike, better or worse, stronger or weaker. As Gentner, Holyoak, and Kokinov (2001) point out, analogy, in its most general sense, is the ability to think about relational patterns. The output of such analogical processes can, however, be used to regulate responses in animals and machines by programming them to respond to these comparisons. Emotions and other feeling states can regulate behavior in much the same way that a thermostat regulates temperature, by activating or deactivating preprogrammed responses when certain input data occur. Although the complexity of human emotions is greater than that of other animals, the mechanisms that underlie them are essentially similar.[9]

Most of us do not think of our emotions as sources of information about our relationship with the world, we just experience them without trying to discern the messages they contain. As Mayer (2001) points out, whether we are controlled by our emotions or control them depends on understanding the information they convey. By tuning in to what our feelings are telling us, we can get an idea of what may need to be changed about our life or our beliefs. Ciarrochi, Forgas, and Mayer (2001) refer to the ability to monitor our own and others' emotions, discriminate among them, and use this information to guide our thinking and actions as *emotional intelligence*. People differ greatly, however, in the ability to effectively identify, express, understand, and regulate their feelings. Reflecting on the information our emotions contain enables us to review options and evaluate consequences before acting, as in the proverbial counting to ten before responding to anger. Individuals who have not developed the circuitry needed to do this frequently end up at the mercy of their passions.[10]

PAST, PRESENT, AND FUTURE

Different emotions convey different types of temporal information. Some emotions relate primarily to the present, others to the past, and still others to the future. Current-state emotions are processed in conjunction with the sensory information system we share with other species, while prospective and retrospective ones involve the ability to construct symbolic representations that portray the time periods involved. The sentient experiences we seem to share with most other mammals, such as happiness, sadness, anger, fear, disgust, and surprise, all convey information about the present. These states, which are often referred to as *primary emotions* because of their universality, are recognized by people in every corner of the globe and are evident even in infants and individuals with dementia. They are all accompanied by facial and other bodily expressions that serve to communicate their message to others. Because they can be processed subcortically, primary emotions are able to facilitate rapid responses to potential harm or good fortune.

We can also use our current-state emotions to provide us with information about anticipated events, by envisioning a future state of affairs and experiencing the feelings it elicits. We are, for instance, able to anticipate whether we are likely to be happy, sad, or angry about something that has not yet happened, simply by conjuring it up in our imagination. We can also sense whether or not we would later regret taking a certain course of action or be upset over a particular consequence, and use this information in our decision making. Picturing such scenarios in our mind enables us to access evaluative information about possible actions in a way that cannot be done by just thinking about them. We can imagine how we might feel if we went on a vacation, got married, or landed in jail, and shape our behavior accordingly.

The ability to use emotions to ascertain relevant information about the past, the present, and the future by focusing our conscious attention on those time periods is a distinctively human achievement. *Happiness*, for example, is a present-oriented emotion that indicates a sense of pleasure about our current situation, while *hope* indicates that we anticipate being happy in the future. *Fear* conveys present-oriented information about threats to life and limb, while *anxiety* transmits information about anticipated harm. *Regret* involves imagining a choice that we did not follow and assessing that its outcome would have been better than the one we did pursue. *Disappointment* results when the actual outcome is not as pleasurable as the expected one. *Guilt*, on the other hand, involves a retrospective appraisal that something that was experienced as pleasant should have been experienced as unpleasant, generally because of subsequent moral considerations. *Excitement*, indicating anticipated danger and pleasure, focuses us on the future and the present; and *anger* can signal that things are not as we would like them to be in the past, the present, or the future.[11]

Many of our more fundamental emotions are automatically processed in the limbic system without needing higher cortical appraisal. If the creak on the stairs sounds like a strange footstep when we are alone at night, we instantly register fear before our intellect has had a chance to assess the situation. All of our more complex emotions, however, involve some amount of cognitive appraisal since, in their case, it is the *meaning* we give to incoming data that determines our response. Cognitive appraisals greatly expand the range of emotional information available to us. Feelings of love, fear, or anger can, for instance, be elicited by recalled or anticipated scenarios as much as by present ones, and the information gained from this can be used to help formulate future aspirations. Most of us differ from one another, however, in what makes us happy or sad, worried or afraid, based on how we interpret what is happening to us. Some of us feel happy at the beach or at a pop concert, while others feel happy in the mountains or at the opera. There is, as they say, no accounting for human taste.[12]

Since there are few, if any, innate determinants of what is right or wrong, moral emotions involve the mental appraisal of given acts in relation to a learned system of values. Our moral values are socially derived covenants, such as the Ten Commandments, that our ancestors developed to enable them to live together in increasing numbers. They were initially woven into the various religious frameworks that our forebears developed to help them understand their place in the world, and they receive much of their authority on this basis. The various sanctions used to encourage moral behavior all require some type of cognitive yardstick against which to assess the future consequences of a given act, no matter whether psychological (*guilt*), social (*ostracism*), or spiritual (*damnation*) in nature. Sociopathic individuals and others who have poorly developed representational systems are generally deficient in the emotions that require cognitive appraisal, including moral ones. Like children and others with limited cognitive abilities, they act impulsively and show little sense of guilt or regret—since they mostly have only present-oriented emotions to regulate their behavior.[13]

Esthetic emotions, like those associated with the appreciation of art, music, and beauty, also require cognitive appraisal. It is not clear whether there are any innate determinants of what is esthetically pleasing or distasteful. Although the physical characteristics that men and women find sexually attractive seem to have a genetic basis, other standards of physical beauty vary from culture to culture, as well as from age to age. Just what it is that certain people find so pleasing about a Beethoven symphony, a rock concert, or a Van Gogh painting, or so agreeable about a desert vista, a tranquil garden, or a brilliant sunset is, however, an unfathomable mystery. It is possible that these sensory inputs activate some sort of neuronal pattern that resonates in harmony with one of the brain's own natural rhythms. There is also an acquired aspect to many esthetic experiences, so that an appreciation of Bach or Picasso may require an amount of learned discernment.

PHYSICAL EXPRESSION

Certain emotions are designed to convey information about our emotional state to others. The primary emotions (fear, anger, disgust, surprise, pleasure, and sadness), for example, are expressed and recognized by people in every known culture through typical facial expressions, gestures, and vocalizations. These present-oriented states, which become instantly apparent when we watch television with the sound turned off, are almost certainly part of a nonverbal communication system that preceded the development of spoken language. Emotions that do not have a distinctive communicative component, such as pride, regret, and hope, generally involve a significant amount of cognitive appraisal—which probably indicates a more recent evolutionary origin and explains why they are not shared by other species. Communication through emotional expression undoubtedly played a crucial role in the initial development of human social ties, and it still helps get them started, through the ooh-ing and cooing exchanges that take place between infants and their parents. As Whybrow (1997) observes: "emotion and emotional expression evolved as a pre-verbal system of communication millions of years ago, when our ancestors first began to seek stable sexual partners, herding together for safety and the protection of the young."

Many emotions are also manifested through patterns of autonomic activity that produce characteristic sensations in different parts of the body—captured by expressions such as having a *gut feeling*, a *broken heart*, or a *lump in the throat*. The physiological changes that stressful emotions bring about often involve either an up-regulation of the autonomic nervous system (the *fight-flight* response), which causes the heart to beat and palms to sweat, or a down-regulation (the *conservation-withdrawal* response), which results in decreased energy and diminished vigilance. The type of response that occurs depends on the type of perceived threat: those that we believe we can escape or overcome elicit arousal, while those that are seen as impossible to overcome or escape produce inhibition. Emotions that do not lead to a direct behavioral response, such as boredom, approval, and envy, do not appear to be accompanied by specific autonomic changes.

WHAT DO OTHER ANIMALS FEEL?

Our emotions differ in two significant ways from those of other animals. We have a richer and more diverse range of feelings, and our emotions create the texture of our conscious life in a manner not available to them. While conscious appraisal plays a major role in the human emotional system, sentient responses in other animals are largely automatic, operating without significant evidence of reflective thought. Although mammals and birds constantly scan the environment for clues about what needs to be done to promote their well-being, their emotional reactions are limited to providing information about their current state of affairs. Human emotions, on the other hand, cover a more diverse range of topics and relationships and include past and future time frames.

Darwin (1872) was among the first to point out the continuum between the expression of emotion in humans and in animals. Most vertebrates express several present-oriented feeling states, including fear, anger, pleasure, and sadness. Fear, as he pointed out, is manifested in virtually all mammals by a widening of the eyes and mouth, trembling muscles, hair standing on end, chattering teeth, and loosened sphincters. Animals that are fearful undoubtedly have some type of awareness of this response, much as they have a sentient awareness of pain. Humans have additional communicated emotions, however, that are not shared with other species, such as crying, laughing, and blushing with embarrassment. Although primates and elephants have occasionally been observed weeping when by themselves, they do not appear to use this as a social signal the way we do. We do not, of course, have any way of knowing the kind of feelings other animals actually experience, nor do we have any idea whether insects and other invertebrates experience them at all. A reasonably well-developed central nervous system is probably required to have sentient awareness and to generate responses that are more than automatic reflexes.

PASSION VERSUS REASON

Plato and Aristotle argued that reason was our highest mental function and that it should reign over emotion in the control of our lives. Others have disagreed, pointing out the important ways that emotional and esthetic feelings enrich and give meaning to what we do. The Enlightenment installed impersonal reason over feelings as the answer to the perplexities of human existence, rejecting the blind faith in superstition, tradition and dogma that had prevailed throughout the Middle Ages. But its great optimism about the capacity of knowledge and intellect to improve the human condition was eventually found wanting. Romanticism emerged in the late eighteenth century as a reaction to the Age of Reason, promising passion, heroic triumph, and idealistic strivings that never quite materialized. Bruner (1986) sees the two as distinct modes of cognitive functioning, each of which provides its own way of ordering experience and constructing reality: a *narrative* mode that involves the dramatic telling of stories and a *logico-scientific* one that involves rational thinking and argument. He points out that stories express and conjure up emotional reactions, while logic and pure rationality are emotionally neutral, and he notes how folk tales go far back in human history as a way of imparting knowledge and values to succeeding generations. The debate about the relative merits of cognition and emotion in achieving human happiness still remains unresolved, however, as much in everyday life as in academic discourse.[14]

Emotions are our main source of information about "value"—how good or bad, right or wrong, something seems in relation to our well-being or survival. Reason, a more recent human accomplishment, uses language and symbolic representation to enable us to decide what to do. Calne (1999) notes that reason "has improved *how* we do things, but has not changed *why* we do things." Thinking and feeling are, however, essentially complementary processes, since reason needs to be counterbalanced by emotion's values and emotion by reason's logic. There are many things we probably would not do if we were completely rational, like fall in love, have children, or chase after dreams, even though these can all be sources of great personal satisfaction. There can be disastrous consequences, however, if emotions run too freely, not restrained at all by reason, as in crimes of passion and manic excitement. Super-rational individuals, on the other hand, have little emotional information to guide them about right or wrong and can thus behave in ways that are monstrously inhuman, rationalizing away atrocities, as the doctors at Auschwitz must have done. Computers offer another example of the limitations of pure logic and rationality since they lack the ability to evaluate the significance of what they do. Although they can match humans at intellectual pursuits like chess, they do not become excited if they win or get upset if they lose.[15]

Although our emotional reactions may seem to make no sense at times, especially to others, they reflect how we *perceive* what is happening to us. Even feelings that seem highly irrational have a certain logic of their own, if only we can detect it. Paranoid fears, manic joys, and melancholic depressions all reflect how given individuals perceive and interpret their situations. Optimal functioning involves maintaining a balance among thinking, feeling, and behaving, with each being utilized and integrated with the others in order to guide our behavior appropriately. The relative emphasis we place on each of them depends in part on which aspect of our lives we most value—the more cerebral or the more passionate, the more analytical or the more artistic, the more secular or the more sensual. Our passions, with all of their splendors and sorrows, represent a significant and irreplaceable part of the human experience. As the Dalai Lama and Cutler (1998) point out, "although the purpose of our lives is to achieve happiness, this cannot be accomplished solely through rational, materialistic means."[16]

ONCE MORE, WITH FEELING

Music has a unique ability to express and evoke emotions in humans, although no one knows why certain combinations of sounds make us feel joyful and others make us feel sad. It seems that an innate capacity for rhythmic activity is universal among humans, for it is included in the lives of even the most primitive peoples, generally as an integral part of their religious and ceremonial observances. Music, like language, involves appreciating temporal patterns of sounds and thus requires an appreciation of the passage of time and the development of symbolic representation. We are often unaware of how pervasive music is in our lives. Not only do we tune in regularly to radios, records, CDs, and concerts, but background music sets the emotional tone at the weddings, funerals, religious services, shopping malls, and eating establishments we go to, as well as in the movies, TV shows, and commercials we watch.[17]

Singing and spoken language probably emerged together as our ancestors developed increasing control over their vocalizations. Both likely evolved from the various sounds our ancestors used to convey emotions to each other, some of which still survive today as crying, sighing, laughing, groaning, and the like. One of the main characteristics of music is the way in which it combines sequences of sounds to produce a balance of surprise and predictability. Music that is simple and heavily rhythmic is generally more immediate and visceral in its emotional impact, while music that is relatively complex in structure and melody has a more cerebral appeal that is not as generally accessible, since the response to it requires a degree of cognitive appraisal. Listening to music can focus our attention so completely on the present that we temporarily lose our awareness of other concerns, which may explain why it tends to move us more than the other arts.[18]

A number of claims have been made that music has a beneficial effect on brain development. Shaw (2000), for instance, claims that exposure to music like Mozart's *Sonata for Two Pianos in D Major* improves children's performance on mathematical tests. He contends that understanding how the brain processes music provides an opportunity for studying the way the brain distinguishes between the analytical thinking of verbal logic and the spatiotemporal reasoning of mathematics and chess. Campbell (1997) maintains that music is able to heal the body, strengthen the mind, and unlock the creative spirit, since it can slow down brain waves, affect pulse rate and blood pressure, reduce muscle tension, affect body temperature, and increase endorphin levels. Such claims, even though seemingly exaggerated, raise questions about the unique place music occupies in human affairs, for, although birds and whales communicate with melodic sounds, we are the only truly musical animal. As Darwin commented in *The Descent of Man* (1881), "As neither the enjoyment nor the capacity of producing musical notes are faculties of the least direct use to man in reference to his ordinary habits of life, they must be ranked among the most mysterious with which he is endowed."

Part Three

A Blueprint for Uniqueness

The ability to foresee the consequences of one's
behavior and the ability to understand how entities
interact with each other are foundations on which the
modern world has been built. The development of
these special capacities traces the history of human
biological and cultural evolution and is, to some
extent, recapitulated as every growing child acquires
language, symbolic representation, and the ability to
comprehend the meaning of time.

CHAPTER 8

The Evolution of
Human Behavior

Nature does nothing without a purpose or utility.
—Aristotle

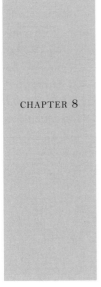Modern-day humans are remarkable creatures, capable of language, abstract thought, religious ritual, culture, and the manipulation of the environment in ways that no other species even remotely approaches. Our brains are the most organizationally complex structures in the universe—three pounds of jelly-like matter that contains billions of intricately connected neurons, each clicking on and off on cue as if in a gigantic symphony. It is little wonder that our ancestors thought we were made in the image of God and occupied the center of the universe. Much of what we consider so extraordinary about our species is, however, of fairly recent origin, not shared by our early ancestors during our evolutionary journey. Notions of hope and despair probably did not dawn on humans until fairly modern times, as they had to await the development of abstract thought and knowledge.[1]

NATURE VERSUS NURTURE

Each of us has a two-fold heritage—a genetic one that is encoded in the DNA we receive from our parents and a cultural one that is passed along to us by the society in which we are raised. Some of the genetic material that we inherit is shared with other mammals, some with other primates, some with other humans, and some is uniquely our own (unless we have an identical twin); the last one is responsible for our individual differences in external features and internal chemistry. Our cultural heritage is comprised of similar components, some common to all cultures, some to our particular one, and some to our own specific family and environment. As Oyama (2000) points out, neither of these inheritances by itself determines how we turn out, since our genes depend on the presence of particular environmental factors to be fully expressed. Both parts of our heritage are essentially informational sets that interact with each other and with what we encounter to determine our behavior—as individuals and as a species. They specify what we *can* do, not what we *will* do, for we need nurturing and experience to fully develop our capacities.

The human evolutionary parade stretches back into an antiquity so distant that it is barely discernible. *Biological evolution*, based on genetic selection, molded the development of the human species for millions of years—from the emergence of the earliest human-like apes about seven million years ago to the appearance of anatomically modern humans about forty thousand years ago. *Cultural evolution*, which involves the nongenetic transmission of acquired information through both spoken and written language, has been the predominant force in humankind's more recent development. It has conveyed an extraordinary adaptability on our species, helping us invent tools, conquer climates, build civilizations, overcome diseases, and develop a kaleidoscope of technological wonders. We are, however, constructed out of exactly the same building materials as the rest of the animal kingdom; our genome differs by only about one percent from that of the chimpanzee. What is unique about us is the way these elements are put together, their order and arrangement.[2]

Biological evolution has come to a virtual halt for us; human survival and selection are now based primarily on cultural innovations. The world we currently live in is, however, vastly different from the one to which we were biologically adapted. As Ornstein and Ehrlich (1989) put it, "the world that made us is different from the world we have made." Although we have created a host of marvels that enable us to prosper in the face of all sorts of environmental adversity, our underlying genetic make-up has not changed appreciably since Stone Age times. Ehrlich (2000) points out that we were hunter-gathers for more than 100,000 generations before we settled in communities some 400 generations ago—which is not enough time for significant genetic changes to have taken place. We are, to some extent, biological misfits living in the relatively artificial environment that our cultural genius has created. There is no guarantee, however, that we will always be able to bend our nature to fit the cultural innovations we create, no guarantee that our great civilizations will be able to sustain themselves any more than others were in the past. We pay a price for our remarkable discoveries, as every advance is accompanied by some type of unintended consequence. Antibiotics save lives but lead to overpopulation, automobiles make us mobile but pollute the environment, and television entertains but numbs our sensibilities.[3]

THE INCREDIBLE JOURNEY

Our earliest ancestors apparently descended from the trees and began to walk upright about seven million years ago, freeing their hands for tools and weapons and setting off our amazing evolutionary journey. The first true humans were relatively brutish beasts who roamed the more tropical climates about two million years ago in small, nomadic bands that lived off the land. Our early forebears continued to evolve over the millennia, developing stone tools, the use of fire, meat-eating habits, improved hunting techniques—and larger brains. Modern men and women arrived on the scene about forty thousand years ago, accompanied by an explosion in tool making and the emergence of cave painting, clothing, decorative beads, and ceremonial practices for burying the dead. The human brain had nearly tripled in size during the preceding two million years and developed the complex information- and language-processing skills that now characterize our species. These early modern humans, who had originated in Africa, lived lives that were probably not very different from those of contemporary hunter-gatherers, such as the Australian Aborigines and the !Kung San of the Kalahari Desert. Diamond (1992) observes that all of the various peoples that currently inhabit the earth, no matter how distinct they may appear, originated from these common ancestors, with the differences between them being primarily due to cultural rather than genetic divergence. As he recounts, "New Guineans whose fathers lived in the Stone Age now pilot airplanes, operate computers, and govern a modern state."[4]

The next major change took place about ten thousand years ago, when our ancestors started to domesticate animals and raise crops at the end of the last Ice Age. Settling in one place, rather than moving with the seasons and the food supply, ushered in the dawn of a new era for our species. It enabled people to live together in far greater numbers than ever before, which brought about the development of more complex languages and social structures. It also increased the opportunity for people to accumulate material possessions, such as cattle, grain, and land, which led eventually to barter and trade. These new cultural adaptations allowed our ancestors to develop new skills and new ways of understanding the world that contributed to their growing sense of mastery and self-awareness.

Occupational specialization became possible once our ancestors gave up their nomadic ways. The logistics of nomadic life limit a group's opportunities; the only previous division of labor had been that women acted as gatherers and keepers of the hearth and men as hunters and protectors. Diversification of labor increased, however, as the settled communities grew larger, leading to the emergence of weavers, potters, smiths, and other specialized craftsmen, as well as tribal leaders, shamans, and kings. By allowing individuals to concentrate their efforts on one particular endeavor, specialization resulted in the growth of new types of knowledge—which was then passed on to succeeding generations. Domestication also brought about efficiencies that gave people the time needed to think about abstract and creative matters, as reflected in the production of decorated craft objects that were no longer entirely utilitarian.

As communities grew and prospered, they brought together people from different tribes with different customs and different beliefs. Proto-religions probably began as ways of establishing a system of authority over these larger groupings, with god-kings like those who built the pyramids of Egypt replacing individual tribal chiefs as determiners of appropriate conduct. The first real cities emerged in the Middle East about 7000 BC. They were made possible by the development of shared beliefs and laws that enabled people to live together in ever-larger numbers. Since they were the only places with sufficient diversity of labor to allow for activities that were not directly productive, these early cities became the centers of intellectual growth and excitement, even though the majority of the population still resided in rural settings. Early city-states grew and flourished throughout the known world, only to eventually fall victim to their own success by becoming too large to sustain themselves, unable to grow enough food and supplies or get rid of the wastes they produced.

Ideas and innovations spread from one sovereign state to another through both trade and war, and their legacy was passed along as part of the great well-spring from which our modern civilizations arose. With the development of written languages about six thousand years ago, humankind finally began to emerge from the shadows of prehistory. Writing allowed complex information to be stored outside the human mind and transmitted over distances in space and time. Having written records of events means that we no longer have to rely on archeological finds to learn about the past. The stories of the great civilizations of the ancient world and of the great religions they gave rise to are, however, relatively recent chapters in our remarkable saga, not the introductory ones they were once thought to be.

CULTURAL EVOLUTION

A culture consists essentially of a shared world view, a common set of beliefs that its members hold to be true. It also involves a shared language, a shared history, and a shared mental model of the universe, all of which are passed along from one generation to the next. Because they share a similar assumptive world, people within a given culture can readily understand and communicate with each other. People from different cultures view the world differently, and often misunderstand each other because of this, with each maintaining that theirs is the only correct version. We often do not see our own culture clearly, as it is like a transparent lens through which we see and understand the world. We tend to see the idiosyncrasies of people who have other world views with relative clarity, but not our own.[5]

As our ancestors developed abstract languages with complex sentences and grammar, they became increasingly able to pass learned information from one generation to the next. They were no longer limited to learning from their own experience, but could now learn from the experiences of others as conveyed to them through myth, folk tale, and social custom. Culture is a cumulative process that grows over time, with each successive generation building on the knowledge imparted to it from the preceding ones. As Plotkin (1994) points out, cultural beliefs and customs are subject to a kind of evolution of their own, an ideological survival of the fittest. Although the ideas that are most consistent with the realities of the external world generally tend to endure, the path toward this is not always a smooth one. New ideas are not always welcomed by the prevailing culture, as Galileo found out when he was tried for heresy because he believed that the earth revolved around the sun. There is, nevertheless, a constant revision of the beliefs and ideas that shape a culture as new information accumulates. We only have to look back to our grandparent's generation to see how differently people saw the world just a short while ago. Many of the ideas and concepts that every school child today takes for granted were not available to past generations. Looking back also shows us how resistant some aspects of the culture are to change—especially ones concerned with parochial and superstitious beliefs.

Tomasello (1999) observes that the cultural transmission of learned behaviors also occurs in other animals, as when fledgling birds mimic the species-specific song of their parents, rat pups eat only the foods eaten by their mother, and young chimpanzees learn tool use by watching the practices of adults. But these other animals do not seem able to elaborate further on what has been passed on to them, probably because their transmission of acquired knowledge is through imitation rather than symbolic communication. This greatly limits the repertoire of behaviors that can be acquired and underlines the uniqueness of human cultural evolution.

UNDERSTANDING THE WORLD

Our ancestors' developing capacities for abstract thought enabled them to begin to generate conceptual models of the world. As primitive humans grappled with understanding what they encountered, they gradually began to embroider a tapestry of meanings and relationships to explain the world around them. They puzzled about what caused things to happen, what made rain and lightning occur, where babies came from, and what happened when people died. They concluded initially, among other things, that the earth was flat, the sun was a chariot of fire that rode across the sky each day, and it rained because the gods were weeping. The representational models they developed and passed on to their heirs became more discerning, however, as their life-styles and beliefs became more diversified.[6]

In those early days, everyone lived in a world full of magical spirits and superstitions. They worshiped all manner of gods and idols and explained natural events in terms of supernatural ones—as various omens, portents and mystical happenings. They initially had no frame of reference to guide them as they started to piece together the puzzle that everywhere surrounded them. They painted on an empty canvas, so to speak, filling it in here and there as best they could from their experience and imagination. They developed simple animistic models of the universe in which both living and nonliving objects were understood as being energized by the same sort of intentions and desires and possessed by the same sort of good and evil spirits. These primitive models gave them an increasing ability to understand their world, predict the outcome of their actions, and take greater control of their lives—ingredients from which the early civilizations were built.[7]

As civilizations developed, the mental models of the world that they had created continued to evolve. Natural events, like storms, eclipses, and floods, began to be explained as mechanical phenomena, rather than as the result of magical enchantments. Superstitious and occult beliefs still permeated the conceptual models inherited from earlier times, however, limiting the range of human affairs that could be effectively predicted. Being able to see into the future was recognized as an extremely valuable talent, and people who claimed that they could do this were held in high regard and sought after for advice. History is full of oracles and seers who claimed that they could foretell what would happen through consulting the stars, retreating into trances, or examining the entrails of sacrificed animals.

A great deal of early human thought was governed by magical thinking, a process in which noncausal relationships are assumed to be causal ones. Our early ancestors believed, for instance, that like things produced each other, that effects resembled their causes, and that objects that had once been in contact continued to influence each other at a distance. Even though these were spurious beliefs, this was the beginning of associative thought, of trying to understand the ways in which the parts of the world were interrelated. Magical thinking was also the basis of many of the superstitious and quasi-religious practices that these early cultures thought would ward off evil spirits and bring about good fortune. While much of what they believed seems comical today, the remnants of these superstitious behaviors still remain with us—knocking on wood, not walking under a ladder, carrying a rabbit's foot, reading one's horoscope. Although most people know that these behaviors no longer make sense, many still feel an emotional need to perform them, just in case.[8]

Formal logic and rational thinking began with the Greek philosophers, whose activities heralded an enormous increase in conceptual thought and the first dawning of science. Modern civilizations took root in the fertile soil of Classical times, prospering or retreating during succeeding periods but all the while adding to mankind's growing store of knowledge about the universe. The Renaissance then ushered in our current era of science and discovery and laid the foundation for mankind's coming to understand the general nature of the physical world and the laws that govern it. Copernicus's discovery that the earth rotated around the sun, by defying commonsense experience, opened up the possibility that things might not always be as they seemed. As the result of such breakthroughs, the church gradually conceded its role as the sole custodian of useful knowledge; libraries and universities were established to advance and transmit the growing accumulation of human wisdom and understanding.

THE ORIGIN OF CONSCIOUSNESS

With the development of language, humans could think and talk about things that were not present in their immediate environment. Words could conjure up pictures and ideas independent of what was actually going on and could generate behavior that was not dependent on the here-and-now environment. Cave paintings and written records were the first objects that represented actual communications from the past, not just stories and legends about it. As civilization slowly gained momentum, humans made a transition from being essentially time-bound creatures whose well-being was largely dependent on whatever they encountered, to ones who were able to establish themselves as conscious beings who could control part of their own destiny.

Jaynes (1976) makes a compelling case that the more complex aspects of consciousness do not appear in human history until about 3000 BC. Written records prior to that time portray our ancestors as having little subjective sense of self or free will. The chronicles that have survived from the early Egyptian, Greek, and Mesopotamian civilizations are remarkably consistent in showing that people experienced their own behavior as being controlled by outside forces in the same way, they thought, these forces controlled everything else around them. They believed that human behavior was determined by the sun, the moon, and the stars, or by various spirits and gods. It was not until about 1000 BC that notions of a subjective self began to appear with any consistency in the literature, descriptions of men and women being responsible for determining their own behavior. According to Jaynes, there is no sense that people had a *fully* conscious mind of their own much before that time.[9]

The emergence of consciousness probably depended on the confluence of a number of factors. The crucial step was the development of the requisite neurological structures, which likely occurred in conjunction with increased brain size and the emergence of symbolic language. Another was the increasing division of labor and work efficiency that enabled some of our ancestors to have time for thinking, exploring, studying, and writing, rather than always having to be occupied with the daily necessities of living. The development of complex social structures and the intermingling of different tribes, each with its own rules and words, undoubtedly contributed to the development of the intricate language and representational systems that characterize consciousness. The ability to understand the universe sufficiently to plan and predict events conferred an enormous adaptive advantage on those who possessed it.

Piaget and Inhelder (1969) believe that children go through a kind of Copernican revolution of their own during the first eighteen months of life, in which they move from a completely egocentric position to constructing a reality in which they see themselves as objects among others and begin to understand relationships. According to them, every growing child retraces the developmental history of the species, passing through three distinct stages identified by the way they acquire language skills. Primary representation involves the use of words merely as labels, with the child living exclusively in the present. In secondary representation, which commences at about the age of two, children start to be able to establish relations between objects, refer to the past, and anticipate the future. The final stage begins at about the age of four and involves the development of self-consciousness, the beginning of a sense of time and the ability to spontaneously recall events from the past. This last developmental milestone, which is dependent on the maturation of language and the beginning of symbolic representation, liberates children from their immediate environment so that they can generate ideas of their own, independent of external cues. Memory improves dramatically at this point, as the child now has a way of efficiently internalizing events in the surrounding world—words are no longer simply labels but have instead become symbols.

TRIBES

Our primitive ancestors lived for almost two million years in small, nomadic bands of no more than a few hundred individuals. They grew up and were socialized entirely within their own tribes, members of other tribes being viewed as strangers and potential adversaries. These early tribes were essentially extended kinship groups in which everyone knew everyone and was likely related to them. Although neighboring tribes were probably friendly during times of plenty, even to the point of sharing resources and intermarrying, they could become competitive and fight with each other when resources were scarce. The more aggressive tribes likely prevailed during these times, as did their genes. It is not surprising that our species, as heir to this legacy, is the only one that regularly indulges in lethal aggression against members of its own kind. Violence elsewhere in nature, with all of its gore and drama, usually involves members of one species killing members of another for food or defense. Fights among members of the same species are usually highly ritualized, with dominance and submission gestures but little real damage to the loser.[10]

Humans have been bred over the millennia to be altruistic toward members of their own tribe and potentially aggressive toward members of other ones. The idea of *us* and *them* began early in the human calendar, with individuals from one's own tribe being treated as *friends* and those from other tribes being regarded as *aliens* who could not be trusted. As increasingly effective weapons were developed, tribal aggression became more lethal and victors began killing off the vanquished as a practical way of assuming their territory and their mates. As Darwin (1881) remarked: "A tribe including many members who, from possessing in a high degree the spirit of patriotism, fidelity, obedience, courage, and sympathy, were always ready to aid one another, and to sacrifice themselves for the common good, would be victorious over other tribes and this would be natural selection." One of the reasons human evolution has been particularly rapid in comparison to that of other species may be that tribal warfare accelerated selection by eliminating the genes of those who were not able to develop good fighting skills. The historian Will Durant is reported to have said that there have been only twenty-nine years in all recorded human history during which there was not a war in progress somewhere.[11]

As nomadic tribes became settled and grew, their members had to learn how to live in larger social groups than ever before. Tribal identities became more complicated as different groups merged and intermarried, and the larger groups to which people felt they belonged were no longer just an extended collection of kinfolk. Different tribes banded together to settle given areas or to jointly defend themselves against outside marauders. The twelve tribes of Israel that are said to have founded the Jewish nation some six thousand years ago were likely one such federation. The Ten Commandments may well have been developed as a covenant to establish explicit rules of conduct between the affiliating tribes, with a supreme being taking the part of the supraordinate tribal leader who would enforce them. Previously, each tribe would have had its own gods and rituals, as well as its unique set of rules and taboos. Likewise, it was only when nomadic Arab tribes began to settle in cities about 1,500 years ago that religion entered their lives, with the appearance of Mohammed and the beginning of Islam. It is probably no coincidence that the history of organized religion dates back to the beginning of the times when people first came to live together in complex social structures.[12]

The remnants of our long tribal prehistory are still in our genes. Still present is our need to belong to a group of some sort—a group to which we swear allegiance in return for obtaining a badge of identity and a degree of protection. Tribalism is still alive and well as ethnic groups engage in bloodbaths all around the globe. It is not yet clear whether different ethnic, racial, and religious groups will ever be able to live together in peace without trying to dominate or impose their will on one another. It is also not clear whether people who live in large, diverse nations will be able to find ways of productively organizing themselves without splintering into tribe-like special interest subgroups. The modern rituals we have developed for meeting our tribal needs, like being a member of a religious group, a sports fan, a faithful employee, or a supporter of a particular cause, do not seem to be sufficient, as disaffected people still join cults and urban youth still form gangs. Civilization is but a six-thousand-year-old veneer that has been layered over the long evolutionary journey that shaped our species' basic nature. The greatest threat to our continuation is probably not from an environmental disaster or a straying meteor but from our failing to find ways to subjugate these innate tribal proclivities so that we can live in peace and shared prosperity.[13]

CHAPTER 9

The Gift of Language

Language is the dress of thought.
—Samuel Johnson

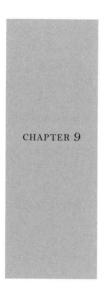

Although we share the same planet with millions of other creatures, we live in a world to which they have no access. We are the only ones whose experience is not bound to the present, so that we are free to think and behave in ways that are not dependent on our current environment. Language is the key that makes all of this possible—for language is not just a method of communication, it is also a means of symbolic representation. The unique way in which it links objects, events, and relationships forms the infrastructure that enables us to understand what we encounter, to reflect on the past, and to dream about the future.[1]

THE SYMBOLIC CODE

Language is a code that transforms objects and relationships into symbols that can be manipulated in the mind and used for communication. It gives us a way of classifying and interpreting our experience, and it shapes the way we see and understand the world. Symbolic information offers an immense advantage over the sensory type of data we share with other animals, as the latter simply records separate events without being able to integrate or analyze them. As Paivio (1986) points out, language contains verbs that link objects (i.e., nouns), adjectives and adverbs that modify their meaning, and endings with past and future tenses, none of which exists as such in the natural world. These linguistic devices substantially increase our capacity for sending and receiving information and enable us to accumulate and transmit knowledge from one generation to the next. Other animals are left to understand the world entirely in terms of their own experience, so that each generation has to begin anew, unable to benefit by what others have already learned.[2]

The language the brain uses to store and process verbal information is, however, not the same one that we use to communicate with each other. The neuronal codes used to process and organize symbolic information represent the common biological substrate on which all of our known languages are built. The thousands of different tongues spoken by people in different cultures are presumably just external manifestations of a common *neuronal language* that stores and processes our internal models of the universe. Pinker (1994) points out how this neuronal language, which he calls *mentalese*, enables us to map our perceptions onto a mental representation system that lets us think, communicate, and make predictions, even in the absence of the objects being considered.[3]

We have little more than a beginning glimpse into how our brains process language. The fact that all of the known languages, including pidgin and sign languages, apparently share the same basic rules of grammar and syntax supports the idea of a common underlying structure. Language functions are predominantly located in the left side of the cerebral cortex—while spatial patterns and emotional expression are primarily on the right side. Injury to these linguistic areas either by trauma or stroke results in various types of aphasia—impairments in comprehending and expressing language. Loritz (1999) points out that the vocal calls of primates, however, are controlled by structures in the brain stem and limbic system, rather than the cortex, the same areas that control emotional vocalizations in humans, such as sobbing and laughing.

WORDS

Words are arbitrary symbols that usually have no direct connection with the objects they represent, which is why there is such a profusion of languages, each with its own arbitrary set of sounds and labels. Words symbolically represent *categories* of things, like *apple* or *car*, rather than specific instances, and then modifiers are attached to describe a particular entity, such as *my uncle's red Buick convertible*. As Bickerton (1990) points out: "language mainly classifies entities (creatures, objects, or ideas) and things that are predicated on such entities (actions, events, states, or processes)." This is an extremely efficient system, as almost any adjective or verb can be applied to almost any noun, not just the one first associated with it. The pliability of these arrangements makes it possible for verbal symbols to be manipulated and combined to represent an endless assortment of objects and events, as well as the relationships that link them.

Words mean different things to different people, however; the more abstract the symbol, the more difficult it is to obtain a consensus about what it means. The meaning we assign to words is also embedded in the contexts in which we encounter them. While it is easy to achieve a consensus about words that represent tangible objects, like *chair* or *banana*, getting agreement about what different people mean when they use abstract terms like *conservative* or *feminist* is more of a problem. The images and emotions that words like *mother* and *police* conjure up also differ from one person to the next, depending on the associations they have to them. One of our major sources of miscommunication is the assumption that others interpret and understand the words we use the same way we do.

Words have always had magical qualities, for naming things makes them seem less mysterious, less frightening. Giving something a name provides us with a sense of having some control over it, a sense that we understand it. Calling something an *accident* or *hypoglycemia*, however, does not in any way help explain it. Primitive people believed that their names were as much a part of them as their hair or their skin, and that finding out people's names gave one power over them. Mentioning the names of the dead or the deities was thus often taboo, as this would invoke their displeasure. Our ancestors also used names to cast spells, since they thought that a name represented its object literally, rather than symbolically. Even today, we often assume that because something has a name it is an actual entity, rather than just an explanatory construct we have devised, such as *conscience* or *intelligence*.

NONVERBAL COMMUNICATION

Members of social species communicate with others of their own kind through various types of nonverbal communication. All of us still retain some of the nonverbal gestures and vocalizations that our ancestors presumably used before they acquired symbolic language. Darwin was fascinated by the expression of emotion in humans: the signs of anger, fear, and joy that can be recognized on our faces. The fact that identical emotional expressions occur in every culture indicates the ancientness of their origin—as also does the observation that chimpanzees seem to smile when they seem happy and frown when they seem perplexed. This universality of nonverbal communication enables people from different cultures to communicate with each other in a rudimentary way, even when they are unable to comprehend each other's spoken language.[4]

Nonverbal communication is used primarily for conveying emotional and socially relevant information, especially when it is of adaptive value for the group. This is why these forms of expression focus heavily on gestures that promote group cohesion and safety. Humans can convey considerable amounts of emotional information nonverbally by modulating the gestures and tone of voice they use when they speak. Nonverbal communication is, however, unable to convey information about the objective features of the world, which is why animals and infants can only communicate how they feel or what they want, not what they know. Nonverbal signs and signals consist of a relatively fixed repertoire and a limited range of topics, varying little from generation to generation. A dog does not have to understand the meaning of the word *come* in order to make the associations that enable it to serve as a signal eliciting approach behavior. Words, on the other hand, represent things symbolically; they do not just name them.

Although a number of species have elaborate systems of nonverbal communication, their vocalizations and gestures are not true languages. Nonverbal communication, since it is limited to what is going on in the here-and-now, is unable to express abstract concepts, refer to the past or the future, or string elements together in novel ways. Gestures can only indicate things in the current environment; they cannot ask about something that is not present or communicate factual knowledge or ideas. Although many other animals communicate with members of their own species through vocalizations, these tend to be stereotyped responses that primarily convey information about their emotional state. They are auditory signals, not symbols. McCrone (1991) believes that, because they do not have symbolic language, other animals live their lives entirely in the present, reacting only to the events that surround them at a particular moment or to memories connected to these events. He states: "We would find animal minds strangely uncluttered. There would not be the same churning of past thoughts and future plans that fill the human mind. There would not be the continuous chatter of our inner voice, not the sudden breaks to reconsider our own actions as we switch from simple awareness to self-awareness." Bickerton (1995) points out that, although domesticated chimpanzees have been taught a vocabulary of several hundred hand signs that denote words, their communications lack the syntactical structure and flexibility of true sentences. He believes that other primates lack the representational system required for these tasks, citing how apes are unable to draw even primitive representations of objects, even though they can readily be taught to produce abstract paintings.[5]

ACQUIRING VERBAL SKILLS

Language is a specialized skill that develops spontaneously in children, without conscious effort or formal instruction. Children in every culture automatically acquire the language to which they are exposed, without having any awareness of its underlying structural rules or logic. It is remarkable how easily youngsters accomplish this, given the complexities of the syntax and grammar involved—especially compared to the difficulties computers have in understanding spoken languages. The way children learn language skills is, in fact, so different from their other forms of learning that Chomsky (1972) maintains we are born with an innate grammar, a specific type of mental organization that makes language acquisition possible. A grammar is simply a set of rules for arranging words in order to convey information. The innate grammar of the brain is, however, not the same as the linguist's grammar, which is simply an articulated theory of the former's structure.[6]

Human infants first communicate through nonverbal gestures and vocalizations, like smiling and crying. They have no concept of cause and effect or any sense of past or future, so everything either just appears or disappears for them, as if by magic. Young infants can only attend to one thing at a time; so they ignore other objects when they are focusing on people, and ignore people when they are attending to something else. Between nine and twelve months, however, they begin to look where adults look and try to get their attention by holding up objects for them to see. These three-way skills, which other primates are not able to accomplish, are thought to be essential for the eventual manipulation of words as part of a way of relating to others. Chimpanzees, when left to their own devices, do not appear to point out objects to other members of their group, hold up things to show them, or intentionally try to teach them new behaviors.[7]

Children tend to utter their first words around the time of their first birthday and begin two-word sentences when they are about eighteen months of age. By the time they are three, they usually have a vocabulary of over a thousand words, make sentences that are seven or eight words long, recollect past experiences, and begin to talk about the future—all of which indicate a beginning level of concept formation and abstraction. The size of the growing child's vocabulary typically increases to the point that they can recognize between five thousand and ten thousand words by five years of age and somewhere between forty-five thousand and sixty thousand words by the time they graduate from high school—although they only use about a third of them in their own speech. They thus learn to recognize, on average, about seven or eight new words every day from birth until about eighteen years of age, a truly remarkable feat.

Reading and writing depend on learning a set of visible linguistic symbols that translate the sounds of spoken words into visual representations. As every school child knows, learning how to interpret these arbitrary shapes is not as easy as acquiring spoken language. This is because reading and writing skills have to be explicitly taught and learned, since we do not have an innate predisposition for acquiring them. As a result, many people in developed countries are still illiterate and some languages still have no written forms of expression. Numbers are yet another system of symbols that have evolved through cultural means and have to be specifically learned. Our ancestors initially counted on their ten fingers—which is the origin of our decimal system—and recorded tallies by notching marks on pieces of wood or bone. There was, of course, little need for complex computational skills before the advent of commerce and science.[8]

IN THE BEGINNING WAS THE WORD

The development of language became possible only after two other major evolutionary transformations had taken place. One was the anatomical modification of the human larynx that began about 200,000 years ago, making the articulation of finely modulated vocalizations possible. The other was the enlargement of the prefrontal area of the brain, which enhanced our ability to process symbolic information, somewhere about 40,000 years ago. Lieberman (1991) points out that we have a longer pharynx than other primates, which is what enables us to make the range of vowel sounds that speech requires. This was accomplished when our voice box descended in our throat during the course of evolution, although it still remains high in the throats of newborns and does not begin to descend until they are about three months old. Because of its lower position, our larynx fails to separate our air passage from our food passage the way it does in other mammals, making us the only ones that cannot breathe and drink at the same time—although suckling newborns can still do this. Just how these evolutionary changes came about is still a mystery; but once language appeared, cultural transmission took over in shaping the linguistic systems that have come to characterize our species.[9]

Language is a relatively recent adaptation that entered into the human drama in its present form probably at about the same time that cave paintings, stone figurines, burial practices, and other symbol-dependent behaviors began to appear. Our ancestors had likely developed sophisticated systems of nonverbal communication during the preceding years, many of which remain with us today. They undoubtedly used complex gestures and vocalizations to organize hunts, share food, establish social bonds, pass on simple tool-making skills, and alert their tribes to danger. The first thoughts that were actually spoken were probably present-oriented two-word combinations similar to those that children first use (*me hungry, boy go, more story*) Bickerton (1990) maintains that these initial utterances were part of a protolanguage that lacked formalized syntactical structure, which took shape gradually over the ensuing millennia. As each tribe invented its own set of words to represent various objects and activities, agreements about usage became necessary when tribes merged or intermarried. Vocabularies thus became increasingly elaborate as settled societies grew and life became more complicated.[10]

The first written languages were hieroglyphic pictures and signs that emerged about six thousand years ago. The traditional way of transmitting custom and culture in earlier times was by word of mouth, with a tribe's rules, legends, and mythology being passed along orally from family members and tribal leaders. Modern alphabetical systems of writing were probably invented by the Canaanites around 1700 BC and subsequently copied by others. Written records eventually came to surpass spoken ones as the major way of imparting accumulated knowledge, but they did not become widespread until the invention of the printing press. We have come a long way since then, with an ever-expanding cascade of words now flooding every aspect of our lives. Language has, without doubt, been the driving force that transformed our Stone Age ancestors into our contemporary selves.[11]

THOUGHT AND LANGUAGE

The controversy over whether thought is possible without language depends largely on how *thought* is defined. If *thinking* refers to any form of information processing by the brain, then it clearly occurs in animals that do not have language. If, on the other hand, it refers to the type of conscious deliberation that enables us to consider situations that are not currently impacting our sensory systems, some form of language seems essential. Bickerton (1995) calls these different types of information processing "on-line" and "off-line" thinking. On-line thinking is limited to processes that connect incoming sensory information and outgoing behavioral responses, while off-line thinking involves the manipulation of representations of words and images that are not related to any current sensory input. On-line thinking is concerned solely with the here-and-now, while off-line thinking enables us to deal with problems that do not immediately confront us—and allows us to generate novel ideas, predict events, and plan future-oriented behaviors.

Conscious thinking, both on-line and off-line, generally takes the form of a verbal self-dialogue about pressing deliberations and reflections, including the rehearsing and editing of imaginary conversations. The main difference between conscious and unconscious thinking is that the former processes actual words while the latter simply processes the neural symbols that underlie them. It is probably impossible to think consciously of ideas and concepts except in words or other symbols. Einstein, who reportedly did not start speaking until he was three years old, said that he thought mostly in pictures, not words. He observed (Einstein, 1954): "The words of the language, as they are written or spoken, do not seem to play any role in my mechanism of thought. The physical entities which seem to serve as elements in thought are certain signs and more or less clear images which can be 'voluntarily' reproduced and combined." Images that can be taken apart and recombined are presumably encoded as symbolic representations.

CHAPTER 10

The Development of Symbolic Thought

The childhood shows the man, as morning shows the day.

—John Milton

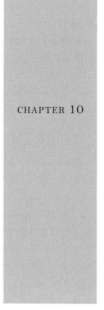

During the first few years of life, every growing child retraces in a truncated and far from exact manner the steps its distant ancestors took in acquiring language and symbolic reasoning skills. Human infants start life immersed entirely in the present, without memory, imagination, or true consciousness to help them make sense out of what they encounter. Unable to recall the past or anticipate the future, they live in an essentially timeless world and communicate through nonverbal gestures and sounds, much as their ancestors did a million years ago. Their developing ability to process symbolic information is the evolutionary step that eventually enables them to escape these age-old confines and assume their modern birthright.[1]

NEURAL INFRASTRUCTURE

Although an adult human brain is three times larger today than it was two million years ago, the size of a newborn's brain is still the same as it was back then. The shape of the human pelvic outlet, the major factor that limits the size of a baby's head at birth, has not changed appreciably since those earlier times. Most of the evolutionary increase in the size of the human brain thus takes place after birth, especially during the first two years of life. A child's brain usually grows from about 350 cubic centimeters at birth to almost 1,000 cubic centimeters by the end of the first year, a remarkable accomplishment even when compared to the other primates. The parts of the human brain that were among the last to develop during our evolutionary journey are also among the last to develop in the growing child; many of them are not yet functional at the time of birth. The neuronal substrate for language and symbolic thought, for instance, only begins to take shape during the latter part of the second year. Prior to that, the infant has no sense of self, no recallable memory, and no ability to think about anyone or anything that is not in its immediate vicinity.[2]

The newborn infant's brain contains almost all of the 100 billion neurons it will possess as an adult, although they must await experiential input to become fully organized and connected with each other. The first neurons begin to appear in the human brain at about forty-two days after conception, after which they grow at an amazing average of about 10,000 per second until they reach their peak at about the twenty-fourth week of pregnancy (Bruer, 1999). The number of synaptic connections between them also grows rapidly, reaching levels that are almost 50 percent higher than adult values during the first few years of life, before eventually being pruned back. Cognitive and behavioral development during the first years of life are determined by the interactions that unfold between the genetically programmed growth of the cerebral cortex and the kinds of sensory input and feedback the infant experiences.

Nature and nurture are inseparable throughout the process of brain development in determining the child's capacities, although experience usually shapes what the child does with them. Genetic endowment and environmental experience are complementary processes, not conflicting ones, for neither produces anything without the other. They work hand-in-hand in evolution to bring about adaptive changes, for it is the phenotypic structures and functions of individuals on which natural selection operates, not their underlying genotypic makeup. Behavior that is usually viewed as innate is thus only so within a particular environmental configuration. As a result, questions about whether brain functions or behaviors are innate or learned are essentially meaningless when applied to individuals. The contributions of nature and nurture to a given function or behavior can, however, have meaning when applied to populations, since the relative contributions of genetic and environmental influences to the variation between individuals can be assessed in discrete populations under given circumstances.[3]

Infants initially live entirely in the present, without any sense of what happened a few moments before or what will happen a few moments later. They exist at the center of their own universe, oblivious to the wants of others and demanding that their needs be gratified immediately. Their behavioral goals are, nonetheless, no different from those of grown-ups: to maximize *feeling good* and minimize *feeling bad*. The things that feel good to them, however, are the built-in biological survival necessities: food, warmth, safety, and relief from discomfort. Even though their communication skills are limited to activities like smiling, crying, and cooing, they soon discover how to use these effectively to get their needs met. The complexity of their behavioral repertoire increases perceptibly during the first eighteen to twenty-four months as they learn ever-new ways of increasing their sense of well-being.

The child progresses through a series of overlapping stages from birth through adolescence. The first six months produce an exploring, socially responsive being who is actively interested in the environment. Infants begin to smile at a human face by about three months of age and "fall in love" with their caregivers as the two respond emotionally to each other. They become distressed when separated from their caregiver from about eight months until they begin to develop a sense of object constancy at about twelve to eighteen months of age. With the onset of symbolic thought, which occurs at this time, there is a realization that mother will return, as well as a beginning sense of self. Two-year-olds are able to generate ideas about things they want to do and implement plans to achieve them, while three-year-olds begin to make genuine causal inferences and appreciate the connections between events. By about their fourth birthday, children begin to talk about mental states in themselves and others and start to experience the inner voices of pride and shame.[4]

Rather than having a large number of specific adaptive behaviors built into our genetic makeup, we have been designed to learn how to cope with the world largely through experience—an evolutionary strategy that enables us to adapt to an extremely wide range of environments. Human infants are unlike other primates in that they are intensely curious about their environment, focus on all sorts of objects in their surroundings, and try to understand the things they encounter. They are biologically programmed to respond to change and novelty, like the movement of an object against a background, rather than to static situations. Once they begin to acquire language, they want to have everything explained to them, and they begin to seek information verbally as well as experientially. Gopnik, Melzoff, and Kuhl (1999) note how young children glean additional information about the world by acting and experimenting on it, rather than just observing it. What they encounter as they grow up, and how they experience it, determines what they eventually come to believe.⁵

Imitative learning is particularly prominent in infants and young children as they watch and mimic all manner of things their parents and siblings do. Morgan (1995) discusses how they learn to interact with others by copying their family members and that they model their attitudes and beliefs in much the same way. A great deal of childhood play involves rehearsing and practicing these imitatively learned roles and behaviors. The capacity for imitative learning decreases with age, however, so that it is significantly reduced by age six and virtually gone by the time of puberty. This may explain why learning a second language as an adult is so difficult. As imitative learning decreases, verbal and intellectual learning take over; and, once this happens, there is usually no holding children back. They begin to express themselves in sentences of ever-increasing complexity, anticipate what will happen, and acquire a growing sense of mastery and accomplishment. They start to experience the world as a series of continuities, rather than as a parade of unrelated episodes, which enables them to begin to work out how things are related—what causes what, what goes with what, and what does not.⁶

A MIRACULOUS TRANSFORMATION

Human infants are gradually transformed during the first three to four years of life from helpless, dependent, tongue-tied, present-oriented creatures into curious, energetic, and articulate youngsters who have ideas and a personality of their own. This metamorphosis, which never fails to amaze those who witness it, mirrors the brain's developing capacity for processing symbolic information. From the very beginning, newborn infants try to make sense out of the myriad of sensory stimuli that impinge on them. As different objects and feelings get recognized and sorted out, they become encoded as distinct patterns of neuronal connectivity. Then, as the brain matures, these sensory representations become complemented by symbolic ones that encode abstract entities, including categories (*dog, toy,* etc.) concepts (*all gone, more,* etc.) and relationships (*on, after, bigger,* etc.) Sigel (1999) concludes that three-year-olds have begun to form representational models, since they can locate a hidden object in a real room after being shown where a miniature replica of it is hidden in a scale model of the room. This is something two-and-a-half-year-olds and non-human primates are not able to do.

The development of language is intimately dependent on the ability to process symbolic information, and its appearance reflects the maturation of the underlying neuronal competency that makes this possible. The first words that children utter just name things, they do not symbolize them. By thirty-six months, however, they can combine words into phrases and sentences that can recount past events and describe anticipated ones. Their language at this stage begins to include abstract parts of speech, such as articles (*the, an*), prepositions (*on, of, it*), and pronouns (*he, she, them*), as well as tenses, plurals, and possessives, none of which is acquired as the result of direct sensory experience. They are all abstractions that do not exist as such in the natural world, linguistic tools that represent the various ways symbolic representations relate to each other.

SYMBOLIC THOUGHT

A number of developmental milestones coincide with the beginning of the child's ability to process symbolic information. While each of these emerges at about the same time, they all have precursors and develop further as the child continues to mature. They include:

- *Object Constancy.* Object constancy involves the realization that people and objects are continuous over time, even when not physically present. Infants initially act as if objects that are not currently being perceived do not exist, indicating that they do not yet have reliable mental representations of them. Up until about nine months, if a toy they have been playing with is temporarily covered by a cloth, they act as if it had never existed; but, shortly after that age, they begin to remove the cloth to retrieve the toy, and several months later do so even when they have been prevented from responding by an interval of several minutes.
- *Cause and Effect.* Although young infants learn to make causal connections about the impact their own actions have on their world, Cullingford (1999) notes that they are not able to appreciate relationships between different external objects until they are about three years old. While their sensory information system can record exter-

nal events, symbolic representations are required to make inferences about the way events are connected and about the passage of time. These skills are, of course, prerequisites for appreciating cause and effect relationships.

• *Sense of Self and Others.* The sense of one's self as an independent entity usually commences at about twelve to eighteen months as youngsters begin to appreciate their own object constancy, as well as that of others. While children can recognize themselves in a mirror by age two, they do not develop a coherent mental representation of themselves until they are about four, roughly the time that they begin to be able to recall past events and establish an awareness of time. As their experiences and competencies grow, their self-representations are enhanced, which reflects their growing awareness of their own needs, aspirations, and values. Tomasello (1999) believes that the ability to understand oneself and others as intentional agents is the critical evolutionary change that differentiated humans from the other primates.[7]

• *Categorical Thinking.* While sensory representations encode real-life events, symbolic ones encode abstract classes of objects and the relationships between them. Symbolic representations are stored and catalogued in clusters of like objects—categories that contain functionally equivalent entities that do not need to be differentiated for purposes of understanding and model building. The category *automobile,* for instance, contains an assorted group of objects that share a similar function and generally predictable outcome. Categorization is an example of how symbolic representations are organized to form a working model of the universe, each representation eventually being linked to others within a hierarchical system.[8]

• *Pride, Shame, and Guilt.* Sometime after the middle of the second year, children begin to develop standards of what is good and what is bad, allowed or not allowed in the world they inhabit. The beginning feelings of pride, shame, and guilt that emerge during this time depend on the development of symbolic representations of the right and wrong way of behaving in given situations. Three-year-olds are still protected from feeling guilty when they break something because they have no conception that the act could have been avoided. By the time they are six, however, their self-representation includes the belief that they have a degree of choice over what they do, a sense of free will—which is the basis of moral behavior. Kagan (1984) believes that "the capacity to evaluate the actions of self and others as good or bad is one of the psychological qualities that most distinguishes *Homo sapiens* from the higher apes."[9]

DEVELOPING A MODEL

Healthy young children begin to develop representational models of the world by about two years of age, based on what they have so far encountered. They continue to embellish and refine these models as their range of experience keeps expanding during their formative years. The models young children build consist initially of unconnected clusters of information, like the first connections in assembling a puzzle. These clusters then start to coalesce into a more unified model by about six years of age, the time that the child begins to understand abstract rules and make deductive inferences. The accuracy of the models they build depends, of course, on how closely the information on which they are based samples the real world. The constructs growing children have of themselves include a variety of dimensions that are based on their interactions with the adults who take care of them, including their beginning concepts of self-esteem, self-confidence, and self-effectiveness. All of these play a major role in determining how secure children feel and how actively they explore the world around them.[10]

Children's lives have to be filled with moderately stimulating and reasonably consistent experiences in order for them to be able to construct a coherent model of the world in which they live. New experiences are best introduced in a gradual and orderly fashion, so that they can adapt and master the changes involved. Where possible, emotional arousal during early development should be kept to a manageable intensity in order to protect the child from being overwhelmed. It is important, however, to distinguish between the amount of stimulation a child receives and the amount of information an experience contains. Large amounts of chaotic, unstructured stimulation contain little usable information for the developing youngster. The child's model of the world has to be built gradually, one construct at a time, like a set of building blocks. The developing brain needs to experience both sufficient constancy and sufficient variation, with the former acting as a background against which sense can be made of the latter.[11]

LEARNING WHAT TO EXPECT

Just like all of nature's other creatures, human infants start life completely in the present, because their nervous systems have not yet developed sufficiently to have a sense of the past or the future. They are unable even to conceive of the possibility of deferring gratification—they simply want what they want when they want it. The capacity to generate expectations about the out-of-sight future has to wait until they are able to process symbolic information. As their experiences accumulate and their models start to take shape, growing children begin to anticipate what is likely to happen within familiar situations. With time and a supportive environment, they eventually realize they do not need to have all of their needs met instantly, that good things will come if they wait and behave appropriately.

Growing infants need to be exposed to a relatively structured environment that they can depend on in order to develop the ability to anticipate events. They should have relatively consistent routines, caregivers, foods, crib times, light cycles, adventitious noises, and the like, for it is only against such a background that orderly changes can be registered. Young children who grow up in extremely disorganized or impoverished environments are less able to perceive patterns in the universe, and thus less able to predict what is likely to happen. Everything is like noise to them, random events that have little relation to each other. Not being able to appreciate the longer-term consequences of their actions, they tend to become prisoners of the here-and-now, with little to counterbalance the pull of their impulses. Therefore, as they grow up they are particularly susceptible to the instant gratification associated with substance abuse and antisocial behavior. Greenspan (1997) maintains, "We can expect that persons who in childhood lacked opportunities to develop higher, more reflective mental qualities will act impulsively, think in rigid and polarized terms, fall short in nuance and subtlety, and ignore the rights, needs and dignity of others." He is concerned that if the numbers of such people grow, society will become more unpredictable and dangerous, with rising levels of violence and antisocial behavior.[12]

Although much of what growing children become is determined by their genetic blueprint, they need to be held, nurtured, and loved to develop their full physical and mental potentials. They also need to be spoken to and interacted with on a regular basis to fully develop their language and intellectual capabilities. Infants who do not develop a secure sense of attachment to their caregivers exhibit a noticeable timidity in exploring the world and tend to grow up feeling fearful and insecure. Children who experience significant amounts of inconsistency in the world around them grow up with a lack of confidence in themselves and a decreased ability to anticipate the future. Ones who are regularly belittled, shamed, rejected, or abused by their parents tend to incorporate these experiences into their developing self-concept—by thinking of themselves as inadequate or un-lovable. Although a child's family may fall short in many ways, the minds of growing children are relatively forgiving of minor insults. They also get exposed eventually to other formative influences, such as schools, churches, and friends, which provide differing views that can modify their earlier beliefs and self-concepts.[13]

SOCIALIZATION AND ENCULTURATION

Human infants acquire their sociocultural heritage through exposure to the overlapping processes of socialization and enculturation. Socialization involves learning the rules for interacting appropriately with and respect-ing the rights of other individuals, both friends and strangers. Humans are socialized first to their family, then to their immediate kinship group, and then to their larger community. When the tribe was the larger society within which individuals lived out their lives, socialization to the adult social order was virtually guaranteed; but in today's complex societies, a number of individuals grow up relatively unsocialized to the communities in which they live. They have little concern for the rights of their fellow citizens and little internal restraint against exploiting or harming them—which they can do without remorse or compassion.[14]

Enculturation involves learning the accumulated knowledge and wis-dom of one's own people—one's family, tribe, and nation. It determines which language we speak, which religion we embrace, and how we con-ceive of the universe and our place in it. In primitive societies, it involves passing along information about what is good to eat and what is not, which things are helpful and which harmful, and how to grow, gather, or hunt for food. As societies become more complex, enculturation involves learning and assimilating more varied concerns, including the meanings its mem-bers attribute to events and the superstitions, myths, and beliefs they share. The prevailing folkways in modern, technological societies are much more elaborate, even though the rules and customs are often invisible to those who have been brought up in them.

The legacy of accumulated knowledge that today's children inherit is far greater than the one their ancestors received. In more-developed coun-tries, this cultural heritage consists of a mixture of scientific knowledge, pragmatic belief, and family values, all of which help shape the growing child's assumptive world. So-called *feral* children, who have been found after apparently being abandoned and raised by wild animals, do not be-come fully human, no matter how much subsequent education they receive.

What young children pick up, of course, depends on what they are exposed to. They are heirs to all sorts of beliefs, customs, and values, which they initially adopt without question but may subsequently modify as a result of education and experience. Today, much of the information that young children receive about the world is, for better or worse, conveyed by television. Although repeatedly exposing children to sexuality and violence may prepare them for the world they will enter, it may also desensitize them and promote maladaptive behavior. There is no doubt that what young minds are exposed to on television shapes their perception of the world, especially since they tend to imitate so much of what they see and hear.[15]

Psychological development, unlike physical development, proceeds throughout the life cycle. It is shaped by the biological clocks that govern reproduction and aging, as well as by the particular experiences individuals have and the types of learning and knowledge they acquire. Every encounter we have, every relationship we establish, every lesson we learn, every book we read, and every show we watch leaves its trace in shaping our mental models of the world. But, because what comes later is built on what came before, formative experiences during childhood play a major role in molding adult destiny, sometimes in ways that cannot be later modified. Our brains lose their plasticity over time as their cells gradually die off, rendering us less able to develop new ideas and adapt to new circumstances. Thus, hopes that thrive in youth usually need to be exchanged for more realistic aspirations as we proceed through the life cycle.

CHAPTER 11

The Concept of Time

If someone asks me what time is, I know what it is;
but if they ask me to explain it, I do not know.
—St. Augustine

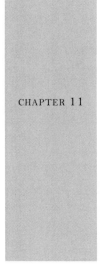

We are the only species that has a true awareness of time, a sense of having a past, a present, and a future. The concept of time is a construct that our ancestors devised to comprehend the orderly changes they found in the universe—the daily cycle of the sun, the recurring phases of the moon, and the annual rhythm of the seasons. Later, they began to use these natural occurrences as yardsticks against which to measure the duration of other events. As our ability to process symbolic information matured, however, our understanding of time gradually changed—and we emerged from the essentially timeless world that characterized the lives of our remote predecessors into one of increasing temporal structure and complexity.[1]

THE GREAT MYSTERY

Time is a phenomenon that still puzzles scientists and philosophers. Our subjective sense of time, which we experience as perceived change against a background of constancy, is not the same as the objective, clock time which we use to measure it. What is more, neither of these helps us understand what time really is or how it began. The instruments we use to measure time, no matter how accurate they seem, are nothing more than devices that change in a highly uniform manner—so that they can be calibrated and standardized in the same way a meter bar can be standardized to measure length. Einstein proposed that all time was relative, since there was no absolutely constant background in the universe against which to measure the occurrence of change. He is reported to have said that time is simply what a clock reads, no matter whether the clock is the rotation of the earth, an hourglass, a pulse count, the thickness of geological deposits, or the measured vibrations of a cesium atom.[2]

Time, in fact, has no clear meaning unless a sequence of events is observed by an individual or a machine at a certain location in the universe. It is not something that we experience directly, but something we *infer* from our experience of the order in which events occur. The only thing our sensory apparatus actually *experiences* is that events occur either simultaneously or in succession, with an interval of varying length between them. The symbolic system then *organizes* these experiences by encoding their temporal relationships. This is something the sensory system is unable to do, which is why animals and young children do not experience the passage of time the way we do. Symbolic representations also calibrate the duration between successive events, so that we can make estimates of how long ago something happened or when something is likely to take place in the future. Our sense of time is essentially a product of human consciousness, for temporal sequencing requires information to be processed in the same serial manner that makes language and rational thought possible.[3]

Despite all of our other advances, the concept of time remains an enigma. The idea that it does not exist independent of an observer challenges our commonsense experience of it. Al-Azm (1967) mentions how Kant (1724–1804) identified the problem: "If time is infinite, it has no beginning, which is difficult to comprehend; but if it is finite, it does have a beginning, which is equally difficult to comprehend, because what came before it?" Heidegger (1924) observes that "time persists merely as a consequence of the events taking place in it." However, Sharp (1981) declares: "Time is a mystery. It cannot be tied down by a definition or confined inside a formula. Like gravity, it is a phenomenon that we can experience but cannot understand. We are aware of the aging of our bodies, of the effects of the movements of our planet, and of the ticking of the clock. We learn a little about what we call the past and we know that change is built into our lives. But neither philosopher nor scientist has been able to analyze and explain all of the meaning of time."[4]

Our early ancestors had only a limited concept of time. They had no calendars or ways of marking the passage of time other than their own memories and the legends their elders had passed on to them. Very young children, having no sense of time, do not really understand what *later* and *tomorrow* mean. By the time they are about four, however, past and future tenses begin to make sense to them, although they usually do not begin to understand the concept of "telling time" or learn to do it until they are six or seven. Many surviving preliterate societies do not share our particular sense of time. Traditional Navaho and Hopi Indians, for instance, have no sense of the future—the only real time to them is the here-and-now present (Hall, 1983). Societies that do not experience the past and the future the way we do, tend to live in a timeless world in which the future is seen simply as an unchanging extension of the past. Our industrialized societies, on the other hand, have perhaps become too time-conscious. We live by the clock, synchronizing our activities with it and eating and sleeping at scheduled times rather than when we feel hungry or tired, as our nomadic ancestors did. Time has even become a valued commodity that can be spent, saved, or wasted.[5]

Our sense of time is linked to our ability to process symbolic information and represent the order and sequence of events. Since none of our sensory organs can directly experience the passage of time, we infer it from our personal sense of continuity. Our perception is that time flows evenly and continuously from the past through the present into the future—and that it always has done this and always will. Experiences that focus our attention exclusively on the present are, however, not accompanied by a sense of time, for we are able to *experience* time only by remembering the past and anticipating the future. We would not be able to sense the *passage* of time if we could not escape from the immediate present, in much the same way we are unable to feel the motion of the earth as it hurtles through space or sense the force of gravity as it weighs down on us. To actually *experience* time, we have to be able to step outside its ever-moving flow. As James (1890) put it: "the *experience* of time cannot simply be explained on the basis of our perception of the world: a succession of feelings, in and of itself, is not a feeling of succession."[6]

Although we conceive of time as flowing evenly, our subjective experience of it is subject to distortions. Some events seem to take longer than clock time (*a watched pot never boils*), while others seem to take less (*time flies when you are having fun*). As James (1890) observes: "In general, a time filled with varied and interesting experiences seems short in passing, but long as we look back. On the other hand, a tract of time empty of experience seems long in passing, but in retrospect short." Because our sensory memories do not have time sequences directly encoded into them, it may take a while to locate the time during which a recognized object was previously encountered. Our memories of the time when past events occurred are usually cataloged by how close they were to some major life event. This is why the sequence of our memories often gets jumbled and why the passage of time is generally experienced in terms of events, not years. We usually leave a remembered time-trail behind us to help us stay oriented to where we are and why we are there, like the fairy tale children who left a trail of pebbles so they could retrace their steps. Having this continuity disrupted, as sometimes occurs for a moment on waking up in an unfamiliar setting, can be extremely disconcerting. This sense of temporal continuity is one of the first things lost in states of delirium, which is why this is such a frightening experience.

We conceive of the past and the future as an unbroken continuum and think of what is yet to come as a logical extension of what has gone before. We initially think that past history is something that is immutably fixed, only to find out later that it is being continually revised and rewritten. A new book on the Civil War or Western Civilization can alter how we look at the past and, as a consequence, change how we see the future. Our personal horizons are similarly limited by the way we piece together and understand our past accomplishments and disappointments. Viorst (1986) points out that many of the changes involved in successfully negotiating life's stages require correcting and revising our life stories so that we can proceed to the next level. Novey (1968) reasons in a similar way that psychotherapy is just a specialized way of helping people revisit and rewrite their own personal histories, so that they can remove the distortions and conflicts that limit the way they see themselves and their prospects. Our past is prologue to our future, although it does not necessarily foretell our destiny.[7]

MEASURING TIME

The notion of *time* as measured by clocks and calendars only gradually dawned on our ancestors. The first functional calendars were introduced almost five thousand years ago by the ancient Egyptians after they had learned to record the movements of the sun, the moon, and the planets.

The problem in measuring time by these naturally occurring events is how to neatly fit the moon's 28½ day cycle around the earth into the 365¼ days that it takes for the earth to complete its rotation around the sun—and allow the dates and the seasons to remain in harmony year after year. Our modern way of doing this was begun by the Romans, although their calendars had only ten months of about 30 days each until Julius Caesar adjusted the total to 365 days and added leap years in 46 BC. This new calendar still lost one day every 128 years, which eventually began to make religious holidays and seasonal events occur at the wrong time of year. Pope Gregory XIII finally corrected this in 1582 by dropping ten days from that year's calendar and adjusting the leap years.[8]

The Gregorian calendar was quickly adopted by the Catholic countries in Europe, although resisted by the Protestant ones. Many people initially thought that the Catholic church was trying to rob them and foreshorten their lives by ten days with the reforms. Great Britain, for instance, did not adopt the Gregorian calendar until 1752; its people continued to live with the old Julian one for almost two hundred years. When the change was eventually adopted, there were riots, because some people believed that they were going to lose eleven days of pay. Stille (2002) notes that China did not adopt the Gregorian calendar and the Western view of time until 1911. The traditional Chinese view, which provided a remarkable sense of continuity for its people for about 3,500 years, was based on a cyclical concept of time. The Orthodox Churches in Greece and Russia did not adopt the Gregorian reforms until 1923.

The Egyptians also developed sundials and water clocks, which estimated the time of day. The first workable mechanical clocks were devised in the thirteenth century, and these were accurate enough by the fourteenth century to be built into cathedral towers and public squares. Personal clocks and watches appeared about two centuries later and initially were owned only by the very wealthy. Knowing the time with any degree of precision was not of great importance to most people before the Industrial Revolution, for their day began at dawn and ended at dusk, with noon simply being when the sun was at its highest point in the sky. The development of precise mechanical clocks in the seventeenth century was, however, a momentous advance. Whereas the hours measured by sundials varied in length according to the season and the latitude, the time told by mechanical clocks was consistent over space and time, independent of extraneous factors. Because these new instruments so clearly dissociated time from natural events, they changed the concept of time itself, as well as our view of the universe. The idea that time could somehow be independent of our experience of it helped create the concept of the universe as a gigantic and predictable clockwork mechanism, which Newton and his contemporaries so brilliantly elucidated.[9]

The increasing impact that clocks and watches had on society was noted by Jonathan Swift in 1726 in *Gulliver's Travels* (Trivers, 1985). The Lilliputians were very puzzled by the fob-watch they found in Gulliver's pocket, and commented that: "It is either some unknown animal, or the god that he worships; but we are more inclined to the latter opinion, because he assured us (if we understood him right, for he expresses himself very imperfectly), that he seldom did anything without consulting it. He called it his oracle and said it pointed out the time for every action of his life." Shapin (1996) maintains that the *clock*, more than any other mechanical construction, became the model for understanding the workings of the universe. The fact that machines could act *like* purposive agents led people to realize that other complex phenomena in the universe that appeared to be purposive could also be explained in terms of mechanical causes and effects. This was in sharp contrast with the animistic view of the world that had been passed down from Aristotle, in which all animate (and many inanimate objects) were endowed with inherent purposes and intentions in order to explain their behavior.[10]

HOW THE CONCEPT OF TIME HAS CHANGED

Until about the middle of the seventeenth century, most people simply believed that the world had always existed as it was—and that it would always continue to do so in exactly the same way. They thought that the entire universe had been created as it was then, with everything being static and fixed from the beginning of time, and that God had ordained it so. The idea that things might have been different in the past or could be different in the future simply did not occur to them. Some groups also thought that time was cyclical and that all of the events that had happened in the past would happen again in the future—which is why they believed in reincarnation. Since in their view everything was preordained, there was little choice but to learn to accept things as they were and wait for the coming of a messiah. The idea that people could do something to change their circumstances was simply not part of the way they saw the world. If their lot was not a happy one, the only positive future they could imagine was in some sort of heavenly afterlife.[11]

Throughout most of human history, people believed that their way of life was as immutable as everything else they came across. During the

Middle Ages, the church even asserted that the very thought that the world could be improved was an affront to God's work. Since no one could even imagine anything being different, Western civilization was shackled for centuries with pessimism and a belief that the Apocalypse was near. Life for the vast majority of people was generally a burden that simply had to be endured, often with drudgery, ill health, and misery—for the feudal world allowed kings and churches to impose their will freely on their subjects. There were exceptions, of course, times when people thrived and looked forward to the future, such as at the height of the great Greek, Roman, and Arabic civilizations. But the circumstances of most human beings throughout history gave them good reason to believe that paradise had either occurred at some time in the past or was yet to come.[12]

The belief that the universe was an essentially static enterprise was the logical outcome of what our ancestors personally experienced and what had been passed down to them. It made sense to them that the world had been created entirely in its current form through a series of divine actions. As Gell (1992) observes, the sense of time in individuals is largely determined by the rate of change they experience during their lifetime; when their way of life differs little from that of their parents and grandparents, they tend to have no reason to think that the future could be different. Until fairly recently, most scholars believed that the universe was only about five thousand years old, the biblical time frame of the Book of Genesis. The true magnitude of the earth's age was not realized until the middle of the eighteenth century, when fossils of extinct plants and animals began to be discovered in the geologic strata. These discoveries revealed that change and transformation had happened in the past and opened the possibility they could happen again in the future. By the mid-nineteenth century, the history of early civilizations in Egypt and Mesopotamia had been discovered, and shortly thereafter archaeologists began unearthing remnants of prehistoric hominids. Our concepts of time altered as our awareness of the historical record increased and we came to understand the extent of the changes that had occurred over the millennia. As the past started to emerge as an orderly progression from one state to the next, so did the future—which opened up as something that human ingenuity and diligence could shape and change.[13]

THE IDEA OF PROGRESS

As the possibility of future change emerged in the seventeenth and eighteenth centuries, more optimistic views of human existence gradually began to take shape. If the future was not predetermined, mankind was no longer doomed to be a mere passenger on the earth but could act to transform it. Western society became infused with the idea of progress, which ushered in an era in which humans started to actively intervene in the world and rearrange nature. It was an intellectual transformation that saw the rise of modern science and the beginning of purposeful experimentation. Instead of just studying the world in order to understand it, people began to act in ways that were designed to improve it. Curiosity and exploration flourished, and romance emerged in poetry and the arts as virtuosos like Byron and Beethoven expressed this new-found freedom in their work.[14]

According to Bruton (1997), the idea of progress began to emerge as "Western Europeans became able to see that the feudalism under which they lived was not an inevitable condition of their world, that the world could be examined and understood and hence changed. It was possible to examine, to probe, to doubt, to search and learn without so abruptly undermining fundamental beliefs and sources of meaning that the whole process stopped. This then produced a vision that modified views of the world and provided the strength—mental and moral—to act, to pay the price." He observes that "the realization that 'things' could be better" was resisted by those with traditional religious views asserting that mankind's place in the world was to be obedient to a supreme being and not question the authority of spiritual leaders. In parts of the world where that tradition has continued, these changes in attitude and outlook have simply not occurred. Such traditional belief systems still represent a barrier to modernization and economic development.

Science, capitalism, and political emancipation became major social forces as hopeful expectations of the future continued to emerge. The wisdom and authority of the ancients started to give way to logic and rationality, and by the end of the eighteenth century, the conditions of human life no longer seemed immutable. The spread of education and social reform led to the end of feudalism and to the notions of equality and democracy that gave birth to the French and American Revolutions. The concept that things could be better in the future also laid the foundations for modern market capitalism, including Adam Smith's notions about the methods of production, distribution, and exchange. The idea of investing capital and energy in projects in the hope of obtaining a later pay-off did not become possible until people were able to predict the long-range outcomes of their actions.

Our current era is no longer characterized by unbridled optimism about the future. As Rifkin (1987) states, "the modern world of streamlined transportation, instantaneous communication, and time-saving technology was supposed to free us from the dictates of the clock and provide us with increased leisure. Instead there seems never to be enough time. We have become more organized, but less spontaneous and less joyful. We are better prepared to act on the future, but less able to enjoy the present and reflect on the past." Many of the great advances brought about by science and technology have also been found to have adverse long-term consequences. Despite our fancy automobiles and medicines and televisions, there is a growing apprehension about the future. As people begin to realize that nature often exacts a price for the gains that science and technology bring, progress is no longer seen as an unalloyed blessing. Threats of environmental or nuclear disaster make the future seem less hospitable than it once did. Unfortunately, when people become less hopeful about the future, they tend to settle for short-sighted goals, often becoming more cynical and self-centered in the process.

PAST, PRESENT, AND FUTURE

Our ability to escape the confines of the immediate present is not without its price. Being able to recall the past and anticipate the future makes it possible to remember unpleasant memories as easily as pleasant ones and to foresee undesirable outcomes, not just desirable ones. Most of our emotional troubles are, in fact, related to concerns about the past and anxieties about the future, rather than to what is going on at the moment. Even when our day-to-day world is extremely arduous, each *instant* is usually endurable. These instants would soon disappear, of course, if we could not remember them or anticipate that they would continue. Unpleasant circumstances usually become unbearable only when we come to believe that they will persist into the future without the prospect of relief. Loneliness, for instance, can be an unpleasant experience, but people only become really distressed by it when they think that it will last forever, that they will never have any friends, and that it means there must be something terribly wrong with them.[15]

We develop procedures for focusing on the present as ways of temporarily setting our troubles aside. As already discussed, in Chapter 6, these include participating in a variety of recreational activities that focus our attention on the immediate moment, to the exclusion of everything else. Skiing, sailing, tennis, and golf are experienced as pleasurable, for example, partly because of the way they make it difficult for thoughts about the past or the future to intrude into our on-going awareness. Listening to music, reading a book, watching a movie, dancing, riding a roller coaster, and the like, fix our attention on the present in much the same way. Meditative Eastern philosophies that deemphasize the self are similarly associated with a sense of timelessness because of the way they focus attention exclusively on the here-and-now. A number of drugs that are experienced as pleasurable, including alcohol, marihuana, and cocaine, also cause individuals to lose track of time—and forget about yesterday's concerns and tomorrow's apprehensions.[16]

Some people live their lives excessively in the present, while others live theirs excessively in the past or the future. Individuals who become overly involved in present-time diversions are often avoiding other matters that need to be addressed. Those who keep dwelling on the past generally do not want to accept inevitable changes in themselves or the world—and they let their interest and curiosity wither in the process. Those who get overly locked into the future spend their lives endlessly daydreaming about tomorrows that never come or chasing fantasies that never get realized, rather than working to achieve realistic goals. Dealing effectively with the challenges that life presents generally involves finding a balance between the time spent in each of these realms. Even though we can roam through time in our minds as much as we fancy, we need to remember that we live our actual lives in the present. This is where all of our joys and sorrows must eventually be experienced, the place our dreams must be realized and our disappointments faced.

A SCARCE RESOURCE

Economics deals with the way we allocate scarce resources in order to produce desired goods and services. As *time* is the ultimate scarce resource for most of us, the fundamental economic decisions we have to make are largely about how to allocate it to maximize our prospects for a happy and meaningful life. Time is an unusual resource, however, in that it must be spent as it occurs—since we have no way of storing or accumulating it. As Becker (1996) observes, "economic and medical progress have greatly increased length of life, but not the physical flow of time itself, which always restricts everyone to twenty-four hours per day. So, while goods and services have expanded in rich countries, the total time available to consume them has not." The ability to invest time successfully in activities that enhance our future well-being depends on how skillful we are at predicting the outcome of our actions. Hopes are like economic prospects that, if successfully realized, increase our overall sense of well being.

Human capital analysis is an area of economics that is based on the assumption that individuals make decisions by weighing the benefits and costs of various alternative ways of investing their time and effort. Most industrialized societies offer a wide array of ways for people to spend their time. While some of these are directly pleasurable, others are aimed at enhancing future pleasure or countering anticipated unhappiness. They include:[17]

- *Paid Work.* Activities that produce financial resources that can be used to obtain pleasure at a later time, even though they are not necessarily pleasurable themselves.
- *Unpaid Work.* Activities that are expected to produce pleasure or avoid pain at a later time, such as school work, cleaning, cooking, growing produce, commuting, paying bills, shopping, child care, and nursing sick relatives.
- *Maintenance Operations.* Activities that are necessary to maintain health and well-being, such as eating, sleeping, bathing, toileting, dressing, exercise, and healthcare visits.
- *Leisure and Recreation.* Activities that are designed to be pleasurable in themselves, including sports, parties, television, reading, movies, concerts, theater, hobbies, drugs, travel, social interaction, and sex.
- *Spiritual Practices.* Activities such as prayer, meditation, and church, mosque, or synagogue attendance.
- *Diversional Pastimes.* Activities that help pass time in a neutral emotional state, such as daydreaming, napping, and watching certain television shows.[18]

Many people lead lives that have only small amounts of discretionary time to spend on pleasurable activities, because of their actual or perceived circumstances. Misfortune and adversity, such as ill-health, disability, and domestic strife, can also consume precious hours. Although leisure was considered to be an exclusive possession of the upper classes until early in the twentieth century, most people in affluent nations nowadays have a wide variety of leisure activities available to them. It is not clear, however, that the amount of pleasure people experience has increased proportionately, as many have become so accustomed to rushing to save time that they find it difficult to relax and enjoy themselves during leisure-time activities.

Part Four

The Human Condition

The ability to transcend time plays a major role in defining the uniqueness of our species. It has molded the ways that science and religion enable us to understand the universe and forged the social, political, and economic structures that continue to shape our history. Depression and despair, however, are part of the price we pay when our aspirations no longer appear viable. Although our ability to look into the future enables us to dream of a better world, we will have to understand our nature and limitations better than we do so far to make this actually happen.

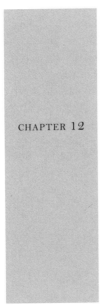

CHAPTER 12

Science and Religion as Ways of Knowing

Lucky is he who is able to understand the cause of things.
—Virgil

Science and religion are systems we have created to help us understand the world and make it more predictable. Each provides an explanatory model of the universe that helps its followers make sense out of things that otherwise seem inexplicable. Heilbroner (1995) observes that "like religion, science was interested in foreseeing the future, but unlike religion, it turned to observation, not inspiration." The basic assumptions in religious systems, which are called dogma, are relatively fixed, while those in science are more open to being challenged. Thus, while religious knowledge is based on revealed truth, scientific knowledge is built on a foundation of experiment and consensus. Because of this, there are many religions, but only one science, each religion being built on a different set of beliefs about the human condition.

Gould (1999) maintains that science and religion are non-overlapping realms he calls *magisteria*, each of which sees the world through its own set of rules: "Science tries to document the factual character of the natural world, and to develop theories that coordinate and explain these facts. Religion, on the other hand, operates in the equally important, but utterly different, realm of human purposes, meanings and values—subjects that the factual domain of science might illuminate, but can never resolve." Einstein (1954) expresses a similar view: "During the last century, there was an unreconcilable conflict between knowledge and belief. The opinion prevailed among advanced minds that it was time that belief should be replaced increasingly by knowledge; belief that did not itself rest on knowledge was superstition, and as such had to be opposed. The weak point of this conception is, however, this, that those convictions which are necessary and determinant for our conduct and judgments cannot be found solely along this solid scientific way. For the scientific method can teach us nothing else beyond how facts are related to, and conditioned by, each other." He claims that "science without religion is lame; religion without science is blind."[1]

THE ROAD TO TRUTH

Neither science nor religion is the road to absolute truth, since both are based on underlying assumptions that are only *believed* to be true. The limits to religion are the more obvious, as the varying beliefs of the different religious systems cannot all be right. If one looks objectively at the various religions, there is little basis for believing why God would favor any one of them over the others. Despite the vehemence they often express, most true believers have simply adopted the religion of their upbringing rather than deciding which one to embrace on their own. Science is also limited, but in a different way. In its attempt to be objective, it has restricted itself to certain ways of knowing and left out ones that do not fit its particular paradigms. Science, at least as it has developed over the past few centuries, is essentially a reductionistic system that explains things in terms of their component parts. It has been spectacularly successful at this—in understanding atoms and electricity and DNA, and so much more. But its success has often bred a kind of arrogance: if something cannot be broken down into components or measured, it cannot be important. Because of this, many of the more meaningful aspects of human experience have been left out of science: love, happiness, and beauty, to name a few. These are private, subjective experiences that cannot be objectively validated—and have thus been left for artists and poets to explore and explain.

There are, however, legitimate ways of knowing and understanding other than those of traditional science. Good art, for example, is the outcome of a disciplined subjectivity that is, in many ways, a counterpoint of the disciplined objectivity that characterizes true science. Most of us blend elements from both of these ways of knowing to help us understand the world, using different models for different purposes. Individuals with greater education and richer formative experiences are apt to favor a more "rational" world view, while those with more limited life experiences are more likely to adopt a "fundamental" belief system. Regardless of our origins, however, we form communities with others largely on the basis of sharing similar views of the world, for this is what enables us to communicate and understand each other. Common systems of belief are what bind us together into workable social and political groups; disparate ones divide and separate us.

Science and religion are both based on beliefs that cannot be disproved. As Couvalis (1997) notes: "The philosophical issues that limit science's ability to directly access the truth are, in fact, little different from those facing us as individuals. We approach the truth through a process of successive approximations. What offers credence to scientific views, as well as to personal ones, is the sense of coherence—the ability of a given theory or view or belief to be consistent with others that have been developed." Religious beliefs are subject to the same test and can change in the face of contrary evidence, although much more reluctantly. The majority of the faithful, for instance, no longer believe that the Bible is literally true, at least not in its entirety. Popper (1965) maintains that "scientific theories are highly informative guesses about the world which although not verifiable (i.e., capable of being shown to be true), can be submitted to severe critical tests. They are serious attempts to discover the truth, even though we do not know, and may perhaps never know, whether they are true or not." The creationists' claim that evolution is only a theory is literally true—for that is all science claims for any of its beliefs, in order to allow for the possibility that subsequent data might modify or disprove them.

REPRESENTATIONAL SYSTEMS

Science and religion are essentially representational systems, alternate mental road maps for understanding the world. Most people try to reconcile the two in order to achieve a workable model of the universe. Religious extremists who are unwilling to make such compromises generally end up with constricted models that limit the areas in which they can function effectively. They are often intolerant not only of the beliefs of other faiths but also of the people who hold them. They see their own way of understanding the world as the right way, God's way, and often feel compelled to eliminate alternative beliefs—as well as those who believe them. The religious wars, crusades, and persecutions that these ideological differences have spawned over the centuries have shaped much of our history and continue to fuel antagonisms in many parts of the world. They bear impressive witness to the power that these fundamental beliefs can have over otherwise reasonable people. Freud (1933) notes: "If one wishes to form a true estimate of the full grandeur of religion, one must keep in mind what it undertakes to do for men. It gives them information about the source and origin of the universe, it assures them of protection and final happiness amid the changing vicissitudes of life, and it guides their thoughts and actions by means of precepts which are backed by the whole force of its authority. It fulfills man's desire for knowledge, doing the same thing that science attempts to accomplish, it assures men of a happy ending and comforts them in their misfortunes (which science cannot do)."

Thus, while science's way of understanding the world has been built on testable hypotheses, religion's views have been fashioned from articles of faith that cannot be objectively verified. Religious assumptions were initially created to fill the void experienced by our early ancestors as they became conscious of their ignorance about the world in which they lived. Their primitive belief systems were largely based on what we now see as superstition—good and bad spirits, rituals, totems, taboos, and the like. The first religious ceremonies commemorated important predictable events, like the cyclic reappearances of the sun, the moon, and the seasons. These early belief systems represent mankind's first attempts to formulate a communally shared view of the world as a more orderly and predictable place, the first steps out of the dark past from which our forebears emerged. Science, religion, and philosophy all developed from these origins, each emerging as a different pathway in our quest to make sense of our universe.[2]

As our ancestors began to find rational explanations for many facets of their day-to-day lives, they no longer needed the animistic and magical systems they had previously used to understand them. Supernatural explanations gave way as natural ones were found for eclipses, floods, earthquakes, and the like. Religion itself also evolved as secular knowledge increased, leaving idols and sacrifices behind in favor of more spiritual theologies. However, the growth of empirical knowledge began to undermine the unquestioned authority the church had previously held over the way people saw the world. The struggles of Galileo exemplify how religious thought eventually yielded to science as the church began to accept the idea that we were not necessarily the centerpiece of creation. The larger questions about the nature of our existence still remain, however, securely in religion's province, as logic and rationality have not yet found a way of dealing with them.[3]

Religious systems have historically been tied closely to political ones, both sharing a history that dates back at least to the first settled communities. The two developed as overlapping ways of providing the social organization that expanding societies needed to regulate the behavior of their citizens. Early states were ruled by godlike kings who had divine rights and wielded absolute power over their subjects, with religious laws like the Ten Commandments also being the laws of the land. The beginning of civil statutes, parliamentary government, and the rights of ordinary citizens did not emerge until relatively recently in the human drama. These democratic ideas represented a radical shift from the autocratic views that dominated human social organization from its earliest days—and still prevail in many less industrialized societies. They signaled a revolutionary change in the way ordinary men and women conceived of their place in the universe. The separation of church and state and the demise of the divine rights of kings left men and women free to develop ideas and beliefs of their own, independent of official doctrines. Democratic ideals liberated Western civilization not only from the religious and political servitude that had prevailed throughout the Middle Ages but also from the rigid intellectual and ideological conformity on which it had been built.[4]

The ideas and beliefs that shape the various political systems that different civilizations have developed are part of the assumptive models their citizens share. This is why universal education is such an integral part of democratic regimes—and repression a necessary instrument of theocratic ones—for to sustain a free and open society, education has to teach people not only what to think, but also how to think, and how to respect the thoughts of those with differing views. Because they do not have this kind of education, cultures with restrictive world views are usually unable to comprehend democratic institutions and thus tend to replace one autocratic system with another when social or economic problems become intolerable. The type of human social organization required to make representative democracies work is based on a set of fundamental beliefs about human rights and responsibilities. The viability of such systems depends on having a common value system that supports open and effective education and a tolerance for diverse beliefs and opinions.[5]

MEANING AND PURPOSE

We search for meaning in what we do in order to make the universe seem more understandable. Frankl (1959) even goes so far as to assert that "man's search for meaning is the primary motivation in his life." We want to believe that the world makes sense, that everything is here for some reason, even if we have to resort at times to magical thinking and intellectual sleight-of-hand to accomplish this. When misfortune befalls us, we wonder whether God is sending us a message or punishing us for past misdeeds, since it is difficult to think such things just happen by chance. Meaning and purpose can only be inferred, however, since the objects and events we experience do not have any intrinsic meaning of their own, at least not that we are able to ascertain. Meaning generally implies that a particular idea or event is consistent with the overall system of understanding we have constructed in our minds, no matter whether a predominantly scientific or religious one.

Because science is purposefully value free, it is of little use in answering moral or ethical questions. Rolston (1987) observes: "Science deals primarily with understanding causes, religion with meanings. Both are ways of providing order and structure to experience. The disposition to interpret things causally and meaningfully are built into the deep structures of the mind; we have to some degree an innate drive to find things intelligible." Russell (1918) notes that science intentionally leaves subjective factors out of its considerations: "The kernel of the scientific outlook is the refusal to regard our own desires, tastes, and interests as affording a key to the understanding of the world. The scientific attitude of mind involves a sweeping away of all other desires in the interests of the desire to know—it involves suppression of hopes and fears, loves and hates, and the whole subjective emotional life, until we become subdued to the material, able to see it frankly, without preconceptions, without bias, without any wish except to see it as it is, and without any belief that it must be determined by some relation, positive or negative, to what we should like it to be, or to what we can easily imagine it to be." This is, of course, an ideal that can never be fully realized.

We seem to have an inbuilt tendency to interpret things we experience as part of a cause and effect relationship. If we see an effect, we infer that there must be a cause, for this is how our information-processing system works. We also infer that if something *causes* something to happen, its *purpose* was to make it happen, implying that an intentional agent has initiated the chain of events. Something must cause the sun to rise and set, the seasons to return, and rain to fall—and allow evil, misfortune, and suffering to occur. But whatever causes these to happen must also have a cause, which itself must have one, and so on through an infinite regression until we reach a *prime mover* that causes everything to happen. Our need for logic and order requires that such an entity exist—and brings us inevitably face to face with some of the metaphysical questions that so perplex us: "How did things get started in the first place? Are we part of some grand design? Is everything merely the result of accident and chance? Is there a point to our existence?"

Science offers us little help in dealing with these questions, for its methods have no way of addressing them. Religion, having no such limitations, rightfully claims this territory as its own. While science's reductionistic approach helps us understand *how* things happen, it does not help us understand *why* they happen. Science focuses on the observable and measurable aspects of human experience, specifying its procedures with the precision needed for others to replicate its results. Religion fills in the valleys and climbs the mountains that science is not able to reach. It provides rules for determining social and ethical behavior and helps us cope with the unknown and the unknowable. Science only goes so far in explaining the human condition, for it is not able to tell us how to behave or make moral decisions. Because science and rationality are cold and impersonal, they offer little comfort to the distressed, little direction about how to lead our lives, little reason to get up and face another day. Faith of some sort is essential for giving our lives a sense of meaning and purpose, no matter whether it is derived from organized religion or from a more personally constructed belief system.

The difference between these two ways of knowing is illustrated by the case of an elderly woman who appeared to be psychotic when she was hospitalized to have her gangrenous foot amputated. She kept asking over and over in a highly agitated manner why her foot had to be cut off. Despite careful and repeated explanations about the way her diabetes had affected the circulation in her foot and the danger that the gangrene would spread, she kept crying out with undiminished fervor. It eventually became apparent that the medical staff had been answering the wrong question. She wanted to know why it was *her* foot that had to be amputated, why it was *her* foot that had the diabetes and the gangrene, and whether this was some sort of message from God. She wanted to know what the meaning of the gangrene was, not its cause. The doctors had given a scientific answer to her question when what she wanted was a spiritual one. She settled down almost immediately after she discussed her concerns with the hospital chaplain—and then underwent the surgery without complication.

Suffering is an essentially human experience that is brought about by how we construe personal misfortunes and the meaning we ascribe to them, rather than by the misfortunes themselves. It involves an expectation that the distressing experience will continue over time without relief—which evokes sensations of dread and despair. Other animals can feel pain and distress, but they do not experience suffering the way we do. Physical pain is a sensory experience that can only be experienced in the present, whereas the mental anguish that characterizes suffering is aroused by the expectation that the misfortune will continue into the future. While pain has a physiological basis that can be explained by science, suffering does not. Science can thus relieve pain, but not suffering; religion, on the other hand, can relieve suffering, but not pain.

Faith has always been our main weapon for comforting those in distress and helping make their lives more bearable. Most of us find that suffering is made more tolerable when we believe we are not alone in our distress, feel supported by others, and find meaning in our sorrow. Religious faith can be deeply shaken, however, when good people become burdened with intolerable adversity. Such events make us wonder why, if everything is the will of a just and merciful God, virtuous individuals are allowed to suffer and evil ones to prosper. Kushner (1989) proposes that one of the main functions of religion is to help people cope with this dilemma: for what is the point of trying to be moral and virtuous if God is indifferent—or if there is no God? He maintains that how people come to terms with this perplexing matter largely defines the nature of their faith.[6]

We are the only moral animal, the only one that possesses a sense of what is right and what is wrong. Our moral precepts are, however, based on faith more than on reason and logic, either faith in God or faith in human nature. We have a mental model of the world that we want to believe is true, a model that includes notions that good deeds will be rewarded, evil will be punished, and justice will prevail. We struggle to keep our beliefs when this does not happen, for we feel lost without them. Even people who are skeptical about religion usually celebrate births, deaths, and marriages with some type of religious ceremony—just to be on the safe side. We are also the only animal that is aware of our own mortality, for the realization that death is our ultimate fate is one of the prices we pay for being able to anticipate the future. It is a bitter pill to swallow, for what is there to look forward to if everything is ultimately in vain; what is the point of leading a moral and ethical life if there is no ultimate judgment to face? All of the organized religions offer ways to address these existential questions in order to ward off the despair that tends otherwise to occur. For some, hope can more easily be maintained if death is seen as a transition into another state, just the end of a mortal phase of existence. Others, however, look more to events in this world for ways of making their aspirations meaningful. The challenge for all of us is to steer a course along which we can generate realistic hopes in the face of the ever-present potential for despair.[7]

CHAPTER 13

Shared Expectations

For him that is joined to all the living, there is hope.
—Ecclesiastes

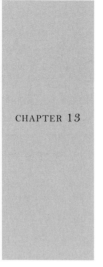We are essentially social creatures who grow up in families and live out our days in communities that enhance our well-being and our survival. Today's complex societies are comprised of an elaborate array of interwoven social, economic, and political institutions that shape the daily content of our lives. Most of us now live in a world in which we are no longer self-sufficient but depend on others to grow our foodstuffs, fashion our clothes, build our houses, protect our safety, and provide our entertainment. The complex structures required to perform these tasks depend on a series of shared hopes and expectations that enable us to work together to achieve common goals. These collective views of the future play a critical role in supporting the modern world by making it a more predictable place in which to live and work.[1]

A SHARED VISION OF THE FUTURE

Communities are groups that have a common heritage, a common belief system, and a common set of values. Their members are connected to one another by a shared vision of the future that enables them to work together to enhance their collective welfare. Most of us are members of several communities—ones related to our work, our ethnic background, our religion, our neighborhood our interests, and so on. These various groups interact and coalesce to form the major institutions that enable people to function as a nation. Because of our underlying diversity, however, we have multiple group loyalties and multiple agendas that can make it difficult for us to work together for the common good—since our special interests often conflict with the interests of the larger community. Because our individual fortunes ultimately depend on the viability of our communal ones, no one profits in the long run if the latter fall apart. When the balance between those who work to improve a community's welfare and those who do not swings too far toward unbridled self-interest, there is a breakdown of the social structure and an increase in deviant behavior.

Family life in today's society is also built on the hopes and expectations that the family members have about each other, just as much as it is on their day-to-day interactions. Good marital relationships depend, for instance, on being able to generate visions of future happiness together—and they fall apart when such hopes no longer seem viable. Parents often invest their hopes in their children and let some of their own well-being ride on how well the youngsters do. Individuals who are unable to defer gratification generally do not do well in long-term relationships, either with spouses or with children, as these usually require a commitment to work for more distant goals. Domestic violence and child abuse are significantly more frequent in present-oriented individuals, since such people are unable to tolerate the short-term frustrations that inevitably occur as part of family life.

According to Delbanco (1999), a nation is held together by the shared hopes of its citizens. He believes that there is an unease in the country when there are no longer any shared hopes to unite its citizens in a common purpose, no longer a shared vision of a better future for the nation. He is among those who claim that the postmodern, postindustrial age is characterized by a sense of emptiness, because "we have cleverly deconstructed our old stories about religion and nationalism but have not yet devised new ones to replace them." Hughes (1993) also discusses the fragmentation he sees in society: "Two hundred and sixty million people make up the same country, but this does not mean that they are all the same kind of people, with the same beliefs and mores. The fact remains that America is a collective work of the imagination, whose making never ends, and once that sense of collectivity and mutual respect is broken, the possibilities of American-ness begin to unravel. If they are fraying now, it is because the politics of ideology has for the last twenty years weakened and in some areas broken the traditional American genius for consensus, for getting along by making up practical compromises to meet real social needs."

Morale is the social equivalent of hope. It involves a shared expectation by the members of a group that they can gain what they want by working together to obtain it. Morale, like hope, energizes a group's members to engage in future-oriented behavior—collaboratively in this case, rather than as individuals. A group's morale rises or falls as its members' shared vision of its future prospects changes. The more they believe they can attain their desired goal, the higher their morale and the harder they will work to achieve it—and vice versa. The team spirit that morale creates helps spur the group's members to success, whether they are a sports team, a business, a community, or a nation. A group's belief that it can achieve what it desires by working together can become a self-fulfilling prophecy, since believing can help make it happen.

Members of groups that have high morale are able to engage in behaviors that can involve significant personal sacrifice, for they believe the outcome will make their effort worthwhile. Some are even willing to lay down their lives for the good of their group. When we feel good about the future prospects of our communities, we build new roads and schools, approve bond issues, pursue higher education, and engage in a variety of other entrepreneurial activities. When the future becomes uncertain, however, such future-oriented behavior diminishes, as we scramble to make the most of our present circumstances. Morale deteriorates when the members of a group no longer see their communal enterprise as continuing to prosper. The unwritten pact to collaborate for the common good only works when everyone believes in it.

Group cohesion is, however, a fragile entity, since the personal interests of the members do not always coincide with those of the group. As Freud (1930) notes: "In every individual the two trends, one towards personal happiness and the other towards unity with the rest of humanity, must contend with each other." For collective action to be effective, each member must trust the others to also do right for the group. This is hard to achieve, especially in loosely knit communities that do not have a shared sense of purpose. Hardin (1968) discusses how private interests can undermine society's interests, especially with regard to such shared resources as the air and water that surround us, since these are easily spoiled by individuals seeking a personal advantage. He quotes Aristotle: "What is common to the greatest number gets the least amount of care. Men pay most attention to what is their own; they care less for what is common." Hardin believes that in order to avoid what he calls the "tragedy of the commons," we need to develop ways of protecting communal resources that are as effective as the laws for protecting private property.[2]

One of the main tasks of leaders is to articulate a credible vision of the future that embodies the hopes and aspirations of their followers. Their job, in fact, is to lead their followers safely *into the future*. Leadership thus involves defining potentially achievable goals that the organization's members would like to attain—and indicating the way they can do this with the resources available to them. Successful leaders raise a group's morale and bolster its members' hopes of achieving their desired goals. The leader's plan of action has to be compatible, however, with the members' beliefs and expectations in order to secure their trust and collaboration. This was how Winston Churchill was able to buoy the sagging spirits of his nation with his words and determination during World War II, lifting their morale, giving them hope, and mobilizing their energies to fight back.[3]

Charismatic leaders are able to mobilize their followers even when the vision of the future they offer does not appear realistically attainable to outsiders. They do this by convincing susceptible individuals to accept their world view, for their conclusions are usually reasonable once one accepts their premises. They are able to mobilize their members' hopes and energies for dubious causes as readily as for worthy ones, as shown by the influence that cult leaders can have over their followers. Brainwashing involves the systematic modification of an individual's representational model by overloading it with highly selective information while excluding other input. Most advertising and political campaigns are also built on promises of a better future—a healthier and more glamorous life or lower taxes and less crime if we use their products or elect their candidates.

Leaders down through the ages have been fascinated by people who could provide them with a plausible view of the future. Fortunetellers, astrologers, augurers, and the like have been employed by rulers for their professed ability to predict what will happen. Today's leaders engage pollsters and think tanks to perform these tasks, although not always with greater success. Leaders need to have a vision of the future and the confidence of their followers that it is realistically attainable. The importance of the leader's role in providing a sense of where the group is headed can become apparent when the leader is suddenly disabled or gone. When President Kennedy was shot, for instance, the whole nation was transfixed by an

Shared Expectations 143

initial wave of panic, as people temporarily lost their sense of security, not knowing what might happen next or what they could still count on.

Modern market capitalism is a future-oriented enterprise that developed in the eighteenth century along with the new ways of thinking about time. It involves owning and accumulating resources that can be invested in projects that are likely to increase in value *over time*. Its complex social choreography comprises private ownership, banks, factories, stores, and markets, all collaborating to produce and distribute goods and services they hope others will want to purchase. Commercial success depends on being able to predict what is likely to happen in the future and being able to act accordingly—the more accurate the forecast, the more likely that the enterprise will succeed. The investment of capital needed to cover the start-up expenses of a new venture and sustain it to the point where it can make a profit on its own is based on future-oriented thinking. Business tycoons, small entrepreneurs, and individual investors do this by using some type of risk-benefit analysis to determine how much of their current assets they are willing to put at risk in the hope of realizing a profit later on. Successful entrepreneurs usually have a talent for identifying the critical variables involved in particular enterprises and using them to develop realistic models for predicting how they are likely to turn out.[4]

Work involves expending time and energy on a present-oriented task that generally is not inherently gratifying in order to obtain something needed or pleasurable later on. In modern market economies, people are usually paid for working and then use their earnings to subsequently obtain things that meet their needs or give them pleasure. As Bruton (1997) points out, however, a job is more than just a means of economic gain. It can also be a major source of accomplishment, of purpose, and of enjoyable interaction outside of the home, all of which qualities embellish its economic motivations. Good employers try to enrich the noneconomic aspects of the jobs they offer in order to be more competitive in attracting high-quality employees. Many of the newer management strategies involve "empowering" employees by increasing their opportunities for personal satisfaction and involvement at the workplace. Most people go to work in the hopes of achieving these nonmonetary rewards in addition to the monetary ones, and the former are often what they miss most when they retire.

Money has no intrinsic value; its worth lies in the fact that it can be exchanged later on for goods and services we want or need. Accumulating enough savings for an emergency, a vacation, an education, or retirement provides a sense of security that makes us feel more optimistic about the future. Most of us try to set some of our income aside for later, rather than spend it all on things that are immediately gratifying: we save, buy real estate, invest in the stock market, purchase insurance, and contribute to retirement plans. Unfortunately, most of the income of people at the lower end of the economy goes for basic necessities, leaving them little to set aside or invest for a better tomorrow. People without discretionary income tend to avoid thinking about the future, for they believe there is little they can do about it.

Nomadic and subsistence peoples have little other than their own labor and energy to invest in the future, for their life style does not allow them to accumulate more than a few rudimentary possessions. Because of this, they have few meaningful ways of trading present activities for enhanced future pleasure. The practices of storing goods and postponing immediate consumption had to wait until our ancestors developed more settled ways of living, when grain and cattle could be stockpiled for future benefit. Most individuals in less developed countries simply lack the resources needed to engage in future-oriented commerce. They live instead in a world of immediacy, where the benefits of their toil are directly available to them. People in today's market economies, on the other hand, are generally able to amass economic assets and improve their future standard of living in a way that is rarely possible in other societies.[5]

Life in industrialized societies thus resembles a series of gambles. We assess our chances of benefiting from investing some of our resources in future-oriented projects rather than spending them in the present. We are more inclined to make long-term investments when we perceive that the world is stable and more predictable, although we still worry that some unforeseen event might spoil our plans. Future-oriented individuals regularly read the paper and listen to the news to find out what they can count on as they project their lives forward. Present-oriented people tend to be less interested in news that is not about immediate events, such as sports or entertainment, as it is of less value to them.

ECONOMIC DEPRESSIONS

Economics is not an exact science, since it is influenced by human beliefs and expectations. The economic market place is built on shared perceptions of the future; people invest their resources in projects they *hope* will increase in value. The price of a company's shares on the stock market is determined by the predictions investors make about its future growth and earnings, based on their evaluation of its past performance and current activity. People tend to invest in a particular enterprise when they *believe* it is likely to increase in value, regardless of the actual state of affairs. Investors who fail to predict the market's future accurately lose some of their assets, while those who correctly foresee it gain additional ones. Shiller (2000) notes that changes in the market are not always justified by a rational evaluation of its worth, since "investors, their confidence and expectations buoyed by past price increases, bid up stock prices further, thereby enticing more investors to do the same, so that the cycle repeats again and again, resulting in an amplified response to the original precipitating factors."

Economic depressions are, in many ways, like clinical ones, as both are associated with a loss of positive expectations about the future. In times of economic prosperity, we feel hopeful about the future and are energized by prospects of good fortune. Times of economic downturn produce the opposite effect, as people become dispirited and despair of improving their circumstances. When we are no longer able to generate hopeful expectations about an enterprise's future, we lose confidence in it and decrease our investments. As people sell off their shares, others take this as a sign that there is going to be a downturn and follow suit, which results in a further drop in market value. Major upturns and downturns in the stock market usually have a snowballing effect that causes them to grow with increasing momentum once they reach a certain level. Franklin Roosevelt's statement that "we have nothing to fear, but fear itself" and his promise of "a chicken in every pot" helped end the Great Depression primarily by raising people's hopes about the future.[6]

Long range predictions of economic activity are notoriously inaccurate because of the complexity of the factors involved, both known and unknown. No matter how much data or understanding we have, emergent and unforeseen events affect how things turn out in ways that could not have been foreseen, even though they may be viewed in hindsight as logical responses to what was going on. Brunner (2000) quotes Alice Rivlin: "The poor showing of the forecasters is not due to any lack of effort or ingenuity. The real problem is that the economic system is extremely complicated, that our own economy is battered by forces outside itself which are inherently unpredictable, such as the weather and foreign wars." Barrow (1998) points out that one of the differences between economic forecasting and weather forecasting is that the former can actually change the economy, while the latter does not change the weather.

CHANGE AND UNCERTAINTY

Because periods of rapid social change do not provide a stable base for predicting where a nation is heading, they are often accompanied by significant shifts in the prevailing view of the future. The hopes raised in Western societies over the past three hundred years have frequently been followed by periods of resignation and despair. Times when the future looks bleak are generally characterized by economic uncertainty, political dissent, interest in the occult, and a wish to recapture the past. When traditional ways of doing things are challenged, many people feel that the world is coming apart, that chaos and moral decay are about to take over. The mood and tempo of the times have always waxed and waned in response to a society's hopes and fears about the future—and they still do. Societal predictions tend, however, to be biased in favor of recent trends over historical ones, a phenomenon that exaggerates the prospects of rosy futures when things have recently been going well and overestimates gloomy ones when they have not.

Cultures evolve over time, rising and eventually falling as they become too rigid and inflexible. When they are unable to respond to new circumstances, the old order inevitably disintegrates and gives way to the new, and what was once radical becomes orthodoxy. Thus, as societies try to adapt to new eventualities, there is a constant tension between change and stability, a discord between conservatives, who want everything to stay the same, and progressives, who want things to be different. Schlesinger (1949) notes this comment by Emerson: "Mankind is divided between the party of Conservatism and the party of Innovation, between the Past and the Future, between Memory and Hope. Neither Memory nor Hope provides by itself an entirely persuasive basis for political action. But the distinction expresses a deep contrast in human temperament and purpose. Some people resent change and others welcome it. Some are satisfied with what we have; others think we can do better." Heilbroner (1995) contends that the optimism that characterized the West from the middle of the nineteenth century until recent times was "an era in which people began to look to the future with confidence, because men and women believed that forces would be working for their betterment, both as individuals and as a collectivity." He believes, however, that a more apprehensive appraisal of the shape of the future has begun to emerge: "The empowering gift of science, the relentless dynamics of the capitalist economy, and the spirit of mass politics still constitute the forces leading us into the future. The difference is that these forces are no longer regarded unambiguously as carriers of progress."[7]

Lasch (1979), discussing how people become self-centered and present-oriented when the future no longer seems promising, makes this comment about the United States in the mid 1970s, right after the Vietnam War: "After the political turmoil of the sixties, Americans have retreated to purely personal preoccupations. Having no hope of bettering their lives in any ways that matter, people have convinced themselves that what matters is psychic self-improvement: getting in touch with their feelings, eating health food, taking lessons in ballet or belly-dancing, immersing themselves in the wisdom of the East, jogging, learning how to 'relate,' and overcoming the 'fear of pleasure.' To live for the moment is the prevailing passion—to live for yourself, not for your predecessors or posterity." He contrasts this with a prior time when "the self-made man, archetypal embodiment of the American dream, owed his advancement to habits of industry, sobriety, moderation, self-discipline, and avoidance of debt. He lived for the future, shunning self-indulgence in favor of patient, painstaking accumulation as long as the collective prospect looked on the whole so bright."

CRIME AND PUNISHMENT

Laws and moral codes tell us what to expect in the way of punishment or sanction if we commit acts that society has deemed unacceptable. In democratic communities, these rules represent a consensus about the types of behavior that people believe will harm the common welfare, most of which involve the imposition of one individual's wants or needs over the wants or needs of others. However, respect for the rights of others generally applies only within a given community—and, in fact, helps define its boundaries. Except in the commission of crimes of passion, most people tend to restrain their aggressive impulses against individuals they see as being like themselves. Moral control over behavior, in contrast to legal control, tends to operate only within the social groups to which individuals feel they belong. The loyalty of those who feel disenfranchised from the larger community is usually only to their fellow gang or cult members, as they feel they have little in common with the rest of society.

Most crimes of violence are perpetrated by present-oriented individuals who are relatively unskilled at predicting the future outcomes of their own or others' actions. Such persons tend to act on impulse or on poorly conceived plans, with little thought about any aftermath. The threat of future punishment serves as a deterrent only for crimes that are premeditated, not for spur-of-the-moment ones committed without regard for their consequences. Violent crimes also tend to be committed by people with little regard for those outside their own particular group, which may be an extremely small one, like a street gang. Because the first few years of life are critical for learning to anticipate consequences and developing empathetic attachments to others, children who do not grow up in a nurturing and predictable environment often end up with representational models that constrain their sphere of identification and confine them to a present-oriented life style.[8]

Crime was not a major social problem until the beginning of industrialization. Before then, most of the population lived in country villages and on farms where there was little outward lawlessness. Everyone knew everyone else and strong communal bonds bound them all together. Punishment was swift, often by shunning and ostracism, which could mean death back when people had a hard time surviving on their own. There was no concept in preindustrial societies of detaining people as punishment, no concept of prisons, and apparently little need for them. With industrialization, however, large numbers of people moved to the cities for employment—which often could not be found. This resulted in the creation of a disenfranchised underclass whose misdeeds soon overwhelmed the local lock-ups. England, rather than building costly prisons, transported its convicts to America, until the United States gained its independence, then sent them to Australia. Today, with nowhere left to send criminals, we are faced with the choice of either building ever more prisons or trying to make such individuals more amenable to the social controls exercised by the larger society, by helping them develop an improved sense of belonging during their formative years.[9]

CHAPTER 14

Despair

He who has never hoped can never despair.
—George Bernard Shaw

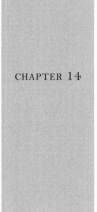

People despair when their life situations are going badly and they have no hope of things ever getting better. They become filled with a sense of futility, resignation, and defeat and see no point in trying or caring any more. Despair is part of the price we pay for learning to base our behavior on hoped-for futures that may not come to pass, for some type of despondency invariably follows when the outcomes we expect no longer seem viable. Grief and depression are manifestations of despair and indicate that something has gone amiss with our expectations about the future. Grief signifies the loss of a circumscribed source of expectations which temporarily disturbs our everyday activities, while depression involves a more pervasive loss of hoped-for eventualities which disrupts our sense of well-being so greatly that we no longer know what to do or where to turn. The various forms of sadness and despair that afflict our spirits and give us pause are, unfortunately, unavoidable parts of the human condition. As Parkes (1972) notes, "the pain of grief is as much part of life as the joy of love; it is perhaps the price we pay for love, the cost of commitment."[1]

FEELING BLUE

We all experience occasional periods of feeling down, when our lives are not going as well as we would like. The word *depression* is, unfortunately, applied to both these normal downs of living as well as the disabling clinical disorder, even though they have little in common. To avoid this confusion, as used here the term *depression* will refer to the clinical condition, *grief* to the response to a specific loss, *sadness* to everyday unhappiness, and *depressed mood* to the negative emotional state that accompanies all of them.[2]

Although we are biologically primed to avoid unpleasant emotions, just as we are to avoid pain and other aversive sensations, they are not without redeeming qualities, for they serve as a major impetus for revising some of the erroneous beliefs we have acquired. As discussed in Chapter 7, our emotions provide us with information about how our lives are going, in order to help us adapt to changes that occur as we go about our daily routines. Sadness and unhappiness are *current-state* emotions that indicate that things are not presently going as we would like. Grief and depression, on the other hand, are *prospective* emotions signifying to us that some or all of our future expectations are no longer attainable and prompting us to review the assumptions on which they were based. As Melges and Bowlby (1969) observe, "prospective affects, such as hope and despair, reflect how a person estimates the probability of his being able to maintain successful plans of action in the pursuit of present and evolving goals." Because there is usually not enough current gratification available to meet our needs, we have to engage in some form of future-oriented behavior in the hope of improving our situation, or we have to accept things as they are, limited though this may be.

Almost everyone in industrialized societies carries positive expectations about the future, both consciously and unconsciously: things they are looking forward to, dreams of future happiness, hopes that things will get better. There is, however, no guarantee that the future will turn out as expected. Whenever an anticipated outcome no longer seems possible, our brain starts to revise those parts of our representational model on which the particular expectation was based. If the impact on our predictive model is circumscribed, as in grief, we are able to retain our unaffected hopes while these revisions are being made. If the problems are widespread, however, the process can completely disrupt our future-oriented behavior. When this happens, our hopes quickly vanish, energy and motivation leave us, and we become depressed—everything is now an effort, nothing is any longer enjoyable, and suicide begins to loom as the only escape.[3]

SADNESS AND APATHY

Sadness, a normal part of everyday living, is characterized by a mildly depressed mood without any change in our future hopes or expectations. It is a response to current upsets or disappointments that do not challenge our representational models. We become sad or unhappy when we believe that our present-oriented wants or needs are not being met, such as when our team loses or we put on weight or it rains during our vacation. Although these disappointments may temporarily color how we see the world, they are not inconsistent with our basic understanding of it and do not disrupt our ability to function. There is little room, however, for mood fluctuations in our highly regimented society, where most everyone is supposed to work and play at the same pace from go to finish seven days a week—like clockwork. We expect people to keep their emotional thermostats set at a constant level, neither too sad nor too happy, no matter what is happening. Less time-conscious societies are much better at tolerating variations in mood and behavior, which is one of their main attractions.[4]

Apathy is an amotivational state caused by the *lack* of hope, not the *loss* of it. It is characterized by settling for one's present lot, rather than trying to improve it by investing one's energy in future-oriented enterprises. It affects people who live their lives in the present without any hoped-for futures to motivate them. They see hoping as too risky a venture, either because of their past experience or because of their current circumstances. Apathetic individuals tend to be withdrawn and unhappy because they have nothing to look forward to, especially if they have no faith-based beliefs to sustain them. They do not become clinically depressed, however, for they have no hoped-for futures to lose. Apathetic individuals numb their emotions to protect themselves from hurt and disappointment—*a-pathy* literally means "without feelings."

Although other animals are unable to predict the longer-term consequences of their actions, they readily learn to expect that a particular behavior will be followed by a particular response. This is the basis of conditioned learning. When a response an animal has come to expect does not occur, the animal's related behaviors go through a process of extinction that can mimic certain aspects of depression. The animal may become hostile and withdrawn, for instance, as it reprograms its present-oriented associations. The dog that sits and whines endlessly for its lost master is presumably upset because its present associations have been disrupted, not some hoped-for future. Animals that have their short-term expectations thwarted can be unhappy or apathetic, as in the *learned helplessness* model described in Chapter 1, but they do not experience the suffering that characterizes depression.

Preverbal infants show similar patterns of protest and withdrawal if their needs and expectations are not met. Archer (1999) points out that children do not experience loss or grief until they have developed a sense of object constancy. They do not understand, for example, that death is irreversible until they are about seven years old, when their concept of time develops. Spitz (1946) found that a number of infants who had been removed from their mothers during the first year of life and placed in a nursery, where their physical needs were met but their emotional ones were neglected, became weepy and withdrawn, averting their faces to ignore people. Many of them then developed a frozen rigidity of expression in which they were wide-eyed, expressionless, frozen, and immobile, as if in a daze. This condition, which he called *anaclitic depression*, appears to be a present-oriented response to emotional deprivation that is not unlike the response to catastrophic loss that can occur in other social mammals.

GRIEF

Grief is a temporary, self-healing response to a specific loss, such as occurs with death, divorce, or abandonment. It can also be triggered by the loss of material possessions or important beliefs, like losing one's savings, or one's job, health, faith, or ideals. Passing through each of the developmental stages of the life cycle involves leaving the previous one behind and grieving over it before we can effectively move on. As Viorst (1986) points out, "we live by losing and letting go. And sooner or later, with more or less pain, we all must come to know that loss is indeed a lifelong human condition. Mourning is the process of adapting to the losses of our life. We mourn the loss of others. But we are also going to mourn the loss of ourselves—of earlier definitions that our images of self depend upon." All of us handle grief in our own way, based on our background and past experience. Some of us have a stiff upper lip and show few outward signs of emotion, while others appear to be consumed by sorrow. But, we all have to come to terms with loss, one way or another, in order to adapt to the changed realities that affect the course of our lives.[5]

The magnitude of the grief response depends on the significance of the loss to the individual. The more meaningful or valued the lost object or relationship, the greater the grief and the more profound the adjustment that has to be made. The impact can be devastating when individuals lose someone or something they have depended on for their own sense of well-being or identity. The intensity of the grief response is also determined by how sudden or unexpected the loss is—which is why it is so much harder to deal with a loss caused by an untimely death or an accident. When the loss is expected, as with someone suffering from a lingering illness, we are able to experience it step by step as their health and vitality wane. While anticipatory grieving can lessen the intensity of the anguish felt when they eventually die, it can also lead to a premature withdrawal from dying individuals, isolating them even more from the support they need. The terminally ill also need to grieve their loss of function and their impending demise, in order to achieve a state of comfort and acceptance about their fate.

The various ways in which a loss affects an individual's model of the world are reworked during the grieving process, one by one, until a revised future is completed and acceptance is achieved. The simplified stages of grieving popularized by Kübler-Ross (1969) illustrate the sequential nature of the response: denial, depression, anger, bargaining, and acceptance. Shock and disbelief are usually the first reactions to major loss, feelings that it cannot be true, that there must be some mistake. As the reality sinks in, anger and despondency descend on the grieving individual, generally in waves interspersed with periods of relative normality. Grief can be such a painful experience, however, that we have to use psychological defenses to prevent it from overwhelming us. These serve as flood-gates that regulate the amount of emotional distress that can be processed at any one time. They become maladaptive, however, when they block out the distress entirely, for the loss has to be dealt with if we are to move on.[6]

The grieving process is concerned with developing an alternate view of the future to replace the one that is no longer viable. The process has been likened to the healing of a physical injury: the wound is raw and painful at first, then less so as the tissues mend, until finally a scar is all that is left to remind us of what happened. Grieving involves repairing a psychological injury—knitting together a revised set of future expectations so that we can again get on with our lives. When grandpa dies, for instance, the grieving process involves going through each of the future scenarios in which our representational model expected him to be present, and mentally reworking them to a tolerable alternative. People who have recently lost loved ones often report expecting to see them in familiar places, only to find themselves suddenly jolted back into reality. Such persisting anticipations illustrate how the grief process involves a one-at-a-time reprogramming of each of our relevant expectations in order to take the full impact of the loss into account. As this process takes its course, the painful feelings begin to diminish and we become less withdrawn.[7]

The nature of the loss experienced in grief helps clarify the mental processes involved. While it may seem that people who are grieving about a loved one's death are grieving their *actual* loss, their accounts indicate that they are really grieving their *future* loss, the loss of the ways they had expected to be involved with the deceased that are no longer possible. The injured man whose damaged leg had to be amputated is not grieving about his lost leg but about the loss of those parts of his anticipated future that depended on getting about with both legs intact. The loss that we mourn in the grief process is the loss of a part of the future that our representational model had expected, either consciously or otherwise. We can only lose and grieve for what we have not yet had, possibilities and potentials that will now not take place, for what we have had still remains with us in memory.

DEPRESSION

Depression is a clinical disorder that affects about a quarter of the U.S. population at least once during their lifetime. The condition is characterized by a loss of interest and enjoyment, a loss of energy, a depressed mood, sleep disturbance, morbid preoccupations, and thoughts of suicide. It varies in intensity, with the more severe forms being accompanied by feelings of intense suffering and despair. Clinical depression is associated with the loss of hope—with the intensity of the hopelessness being the most accurate measure of the condition's severity and the most reliable predictor of suicide. Suicide, of course, represents the ultimate expression of despair, the absolute inability to foresee a tolerable future for oneself. Individuals feel depleted when they lose their prospects of future happiness, as if they have lost their way in life and have nothing left to motivate or energize them. Like the driver who runs into a fog on the expressway, they can no longer see where they are going; they have to slow down and wait for their visibility to improve before they can again get underway. The schematic diagram in Chapter 2 that depicts how hope is generated and lost illustrates how failure along the path to hoped-for goals increases the likelihood of depression.[8]

Although we know that clinical depression is associated with a depletion of certain messenger chemicals in the brain and that it responds to medications that restore these, we do not understand whether the changes in these substances cause the condition or are caused by it. Similarly, while there is good evidence that both genetic and experiential factors predispose certain individuals to depression, we still do not know the mechanisms involved. People with fanciful or unrealistic hopes have an increased risk of becoming depressed; these include many highly creative writers and artists. Individuals who put all of their hopes in one basket, rather than having a diversified range of future goals, are also more vulnerable to depression—because they risk losing everything if something happens to make their expectation no longer seem attainable. People who have been badly hurt by previous losses often defend themselves against becoming hurt again by limiting their future aspirations, so that they do not have so much to lose. These include a variety of pessimists and cynics who live relatively joyless lives with nothing to look forward to. Others defend against depression by trying to fill their time with excessive pleasure-seeking activities, but they usually have to face a day of reckoning when these pursuits eventually fail them.[9]

Minkowski (1933) was one of the first to propose that a foreshortening of future time perspective was one of the main features of clinical depression. A number of others have made similar observations since then. Brown and Harris (1978), for instance, note that "it is the generalization of hopelessness that forms the central core of depression." Melges and Bowlby (1969) report that "the depressed person believes that his plans of action are no longer effective in reaching his continuing and long range goals." Abramson, Metalsky, and Alloy (1988) also observe that "the cause of depression is either that highly desired outcomes are unlikely to occur or that highly aversive outcomes are likely to occur, and that no response in one's repertoire will change the likelihood of these occurrences." Melges (1982) concludes that depression is caused by the "spirals of hopelessness that occur when the person believes that his plans of action are no longer effective for meeting his goals, yet still clings to his goals." Rappaport (1990) concurs that "when the future ceases to be a part of experience, the result is a sense of hopelessness that we call depression." As McGuire and Troisi (1998) point out, "the close correlation between depressed feelings and the sense that life has not turned out as desired is too striking to ignore."

Depression is associated with a down-regulation of a number of physiological systems that is aimed at conserving energy and enhancing survival, the opposite of the up-regulating response that readies us for action. The biological basis of depression involves an adaptive response to stresses that the individual believes can be neither avoided nor overcome—like the hibernation response the grizzly bear uses to cope with oncoming winter. The loss of energy that this down-regulation causes is different from the fatigue *after* exertion that occurs in many other medical conditions. It is an *inertia*, a difficulty in initiating activity that improves once the person gets going, like an old steam locomotive slowly leaving the station. This difficulty in getting energized seems to be due to decreased activity at the neuromuscular endplates that maintain the resting level of muscle tone, such that a larger neural discharge is required to activate them. The decrease in resting muscle tone is apparent in the sagging facial expression and drooping body posture that typically accompany the disorder.[10]

Engel and Schmale (1972) claim that this down-regulation is characterized by a pattern of relative immobility, quiescence, and unresponsiveness to the external environment that is mediated by the parasympathetic nervous system. They believe that this response occurs in virtually every animal species as a protection against certain dangers. Richter (1957), who was interested in the mechanisms involved in "voodoo death," found that rats that had had their whiskers trimmed stopped swimming and died shortly after being placed in a water-filled glass cylinder, while those with intact whiskers did not. Contrary to expectation, he observed that the rats that died showed a slowing of the heart from overstimulation of the parasympathetic nervous system, rather than an acceleration due to sympathetic activation. His findings support Schmale and Engel's (1975) proposal that inhibition and withdrawal, rather than arousal and activation, occur in response to certain insurmountable stresses—and provide a way of explaining many of the physical symptoms that accompany depression.

Cross-cultural studies of depression tend to indicate a significantly lower incidence of the disorder in less developed countries. It is difficult, however, to tell in these surveys whether a given individual is unhappy, apathetic, depressed, or grieving, because depressive states tend to be expressed in different ways in different cultures; each language has its own words for sadness and despair and each culture its own beliefs about them. Nevertheless, it is likely that the incidence of clinical depression really is less in present-oriented societies. Buddhist ideology, for instance, assumes that life is comprised of suffering and sorrow caused by attachment, desire, and craving—the very things that help people in materialistic societies generate hopes. Buddhists believe that the way to attain *nirvana* is by understanding that the world of sense pleasure is illusory and should be renounced in favor of a more contemplative life. As Obeyesekere (1985) observes, hopelessness about oneself and about life in general is an integral part of a Buddhist's understanding of the nature of the world. While that belief helps its adherents achieve a sense of tranquillity by curtailing their desire for worldly pleasure, both in the present and the future, it fosters an acceptance of the status quo that limits their ability to improve their circumstances. It does, however, protect them from the grief and depression that unrealized hopes and expectations can bring about.[11]

MANIA

Mania and elation are states in which a person's positive expectations of the future are so excessively buoyed that they become recklessly energized and euphoric. It is the mirror image of depression. Manic individuals can become so elated and energized that they may not feel the need to eat or sleep for days on end as they pursue a myriad of grandiose, future-oriented activities. Manic behavior is invariably accompanied by pathologically embellished hopes that eventually get dashed, leaving the person depleted and depressed. Manic depressive illness (also known as bipolar disorder) consists of alternating swings between mania and depression, with the suffering experienced during the depressed phase seeming to be payback for the pleasures borrowed during the manic one.

Sustained periods of high spirits are not always pathological, however, although they are almost always associated with enhanced expectations of future pleasure. People who fall in love, have a new baby, or win the lottery become overjoyed by the way these enhance their dreams of future bliss, not just by the change in their immediate circumstances. Romance is also based on hope, on visions of future happiness with one's loved one—the more elaborate the fantasy, the more intense the exhilaration. Some highly successful individuals experience increased energy for long periods without getting depressed afterward, but they are generally motivated by hopes they are realistically able to achieve. People who are successful in predicting the consequences of their own and others' behavior become more self-confident, more energetic, and more willing to take risks. Individuals who are highly successful in one field may, however, be less so in areas in which their mental models are less well articulated.

TREATMENT

Modern treatment methods greatly shorten the duration of depressive episodes and reduce the amount of suffering and personal disruption they cause. Clinical depression is best treated with a combination of antidepressant medication and targeted psychotherapy. Part of the psychological treatment should be directed at restoring hope by helping affected individuals knit together a feasible future for themselves. People who experience repeated episodes of depression usually need maintenance medication to lessen the risk of recurrence, as well as more extensive psychotherapy to deal with their underlying vulnerabilities. Rappaport (1990) believes that such therapy should be directed at helping them achieve a greater coherence between past, present, and future time in order to improve their sense of personal integration. Uncomplicated grief and sadness generally do not need specific treatment, although support, spiritual help, and caring can lessen the suffering involved.

Clinical depression can be thought of as a form of emotional bankruptcy in which individuals have depleted their emotional assets and see no prospect of replenishing them. They feel that they have run out of gas and do not see any way of obtaining new supplies of emotional well-being. Supportive care by family and professionals involves helping them restore balance to their emotional economy by showing concern, helping them set achievable goals, and addressing their negative distortions about themselves and their circumstances, for it is how they view the world that determines how they feel. It is also important to convey positive expectations about the future by reassuring them that their current state will not last forever, as well as by helping them overcome their feelings of inertia by getting them to exercise, even if only at a minimal level at first. Finding ways to get them involved in activities that temporarily focus their attention on the present will provide depressed individuals with relief from the morbid thoughts that otherwise preoccupy them.[12]

A number of the issues involved in resolving grief and depression are illustrated by the 23-year-old electrical linesman who was hospitalized with severe burns after having accidentally sustained a 67,000-volt shock. He survived the initial burn injury only to find out that he had become paraplegic from the accident. He initially responded to this by alternating between completely denying his loss of function, saying that he really could walk if he wanted to, and being profoundly depressed. It turned out that his father had been 79 when he was born, having remarried late in life after already raising another family. He said he had two young sons of his own, aged 2 and 4, and that his lifelong dream was to be the father to them that his own father had never been to him. He was an avid outdoorsman, interested in hunting, fishing, and camping, who lived to be able to take his sons with him on his trips. He realized that this would be impossible if he could not walk, which explains why he responded so catastrophically to his loss. As he began to accept what had happened and think about what he might do about it, his depression gradually lessened. After about three months, he told the staff with obvious relief: "You know, there is more than one way of being a father to boys," and he started to talk about how he could still be a major influence in his sons' lives. He left the hospital shortly thereafter optimistic about the future, planning to open a watch repair business, and determined to get on with his life and his family. Once he was able to devise an alternative, viable future for himself, his depression lifted and he became re-energized.

CHAPTER 15

Human Nature—
It's About Time

> There are many wondrous things,
> And nothing more wondrous than man.
> —Sophocles

Our ability to escape the confines of the present and base our behavior on hopes about the future is one of the most distinctive features of our species. As Emmons (1999) observes, "there is perhaps no characteristic more fundamentally human than the capacity to imagine future outcomes and to devise means to attain them." This has been the engine that shaped the cultures and civilizations we regard as our crowning achievement—and it is the one most likely to preserve them. It is a remarkable skill and one which has helped make us the most adaptable of all creatures, able to survive and prosper in every corner of the globe. It has, unfortunately, also helped make us intolerant and destructive creatures, for despite our many accomplishments, we have not yet found a way to live in peace with each other or avoid despoiling the planet. As we worry about our ability to deal with the threats that confront our way of life, we still know less about ourselves and our underlying nature than we do about the world around us.

Human nature is another of those concepts that everyone understands but no one can quite define. We all have our own mental models of the rules that govern our species' behavior and, although we use them to predict how people will act, we have trouble making them explicit. We think of *human nature* as those aspects of our behavior that we share with other humans but not with our closest primate relatives. But it is not clear exactly what these special human traits are, because they tend to be expressed in various ways in different individuals, in different cultures, during different eras, and so on. There is, as a result, probably no meaningful way of defining human nature, since we all shade the concept to fit our own particular ideological needs. Ehrlich (2000) believes that there is no single set of enduring behavioral predilections that defines human nature, and he argues for replacing the concept by referring instead to human *natures*. He maintains that "the human nature of a Chinese man living in Beijing is somewhat different from the human nature of a Parisian woman." His approach, however, does little to help us understand what is involved.

BEING HUMAN

There is little consensus about what exactly it is about us that makes us *human*, different from all of God's other creatures. Some have thought we are special because we possess reason, have a moral conscience, or an immortal soul, although they have not always been willing to extend these attributes to people of other creeds and nationalities. Those with a more scientific bent have looked to the more explicit aspects of our heritage, such as having language, making tools, and being able to make conscious choices. None of these, however, represents an absolute discontinuity with the rest of the animal kingdom, for chimpanzees make simple tools, other primates seem to have elementary forms of consciousness, and several species have primitive forms of language. Byrne (1995) notes, however, that "the evidence for cognitive abilities reminiscent of those of humans is patchy in apes, even for the well studied chimpanzee." We also possess a number of other distinctive traits, but these are less central to our sense of identity—and may simply have arisen as by-products of more adaptive changes during the course of evolution. We are, for instance, the only animal that has a sense of humor, gets embarrassed about sex, regularly kills members of its own species, is aware of its own mortality, cries and sheds tears, commits suicide, kills its prey before it eats it, and sings and dances to music.

Darwin (1881) upset the established view of things when he proposed in the *Descent of Man* that "the difference in mind between man and higher animals, great as it is, certainly is one of degree and not of kind." Bickerton (1995) notes that "humans are a species produced like all other species by the workings of biological evolution, yet the behavior of humans differs dramatically from that of all other species over a wide variety of parameters. The range of behavior in other creatures does not extend much beyond seeking food, seeking sex, rearing and protecting young, resisting predation, grooming, fighting rivals, exploring and defending territory, and unstructured play. Human beings do all of these things, of course, but they also do math, tap dance, engage in commerce, build boats, play chess, invent novel artifacts, drive vehicles, litigate, draw representationally, and do countless other things that no other species ever did." Kant (1781) declares that the difference between man and the rest of nature is simply that "man is free to choose what he wishes. This, the will, is what enables man to choose between good and evil, right and wrong."[1]

We are also the species that built libraries and traveled to the moon, that developed laws for governing ourselves and medicines for healing illnesses, that produced saints and martyrs, poets and great artists, air conditioning and automobiles, shopping malls and indoor plumbing. Ours is a remarkable history of discovery, of enlightenment, and of achievement—as well as, unfortunately, of violence and brutality. Cruelty and aggression are apparently as much a part of our nature as kindness and solicitude. So-called "civilized" behavior supposedly depends on controlling the more brutish aspects of our nature, on being able to exercise choice over what we do rather than just respond to our instincts. But we are not clear about whether our more enlightened behaviors are part of our underlying nature or merely learned veneers that can all too easily be erased. We like to think, for instance, that people who commit atrocities are not truly human, although we worry that they might be. We simply do not know whether evil people are born that way, learn to be bad, or fail to learn to be good; and thus we do not know whether to punish them, lock them up, or rehabilitate them. As Mandler (1997) points out, the debate about whether we are inherently good natured or bad is probably as old as mankind itself.

Because so much of what we become depends on how we are raised, the experiences we have, and our individual circumstances, it is probably more useful to define human nature in terms of our species' unique capabilities, by what we can do rather than by what we do do. These underlying potentials are shared by all of us—Tibetan monks, Wall Street bankers, and Australian bushmen—for it seems that, under the skin, we are all more alike than otherwise, even the most lowly and disreputable among us. We probably differ more in how we think about human nature than in how we exhibit it. As Horgan (1999) points out, "at their core, every religious creed and sect, every political movement, every economic theory, every philosophical point of view, as well as every behavioral and neuroscience discipline, is based on differing versions of human nature." Although these ideological differences are rarely made explicit, they are evident among the assumptions that shape these fields. They are what makes it so difficult for us to achieve a consensus about policies that address common social problems, such as how much of our taxes should be spent to promote universal health care, remediate delinquents, or lessen the prevalence of child abuse, domestic violence, and drug addiction. For we do not yet understand enough about how these problems arise—whether they are inevitable parts of our nature or aberrations that can be treated or prevented.[2]

NATURE VERSUS NURTURE

Although most people now accept the notion that we are descended from more primitive ancestors, they are less willing to concede that we are simply part of nature, just like all the other creatures. Unfortunately, we have no way of knowing whether or not we have been specially created or whether this is just a fiction we have constructed to make us feel more secure. As Shapin (1996) notes: "We believe that all of the rest of the world can now be explained by natural causes, but we are not sure of our own lives. What if we are only creatures like dogs and horses whose only purpose is to lead out our lives as best we can, to achieve as much happiness and joy as possible while minimizing our pain and suffering." Descartes's solution was to believe that our bodies obeyed the laws of nature like the rest of the universe but that we differed from the other species because we had an immortal soul that enabled us to reason. People who think we have been specially created tend to believe that our future is in the hands of divine Providence, while others see it as being up to us to shape and determine—for if we are not specially created, it is unlikely we will be specially saved.

Current advances in molecular biology promise to shed light on the fundamental genetic blueprint that makes us what we are. Those parts of the human genome that we share with each other but not with our closest primate relatives are certainly one of our defining characteristics. These include the genes that determine our upright posture, prehensile thumb, hair distribution, and unique brain, as well as those that underlie our capacities for tool making, language, and abstraction. We are less sure about the role that genes play in determining our social behavior, or the extent to which they are responsible for our being creative, hateful, idealistic, or industrious. Wilson (1978) believes that our fundamental social and behavioral capacities have been largely shaped by natural selection over the millennia. He maintains that genetic changes that affect social behavior in ways that lead to increased reproductive success have been selected through evolution, even though they may depend on environmental factors to be fully expressed. The interaction between our genetic endowment and the environment in which we develop our capacities is not a simple one, however, as both play a crucial role in the drama that enables us to become fully human.[3]

Our nature is not determined just by our genetic legacy, since it is also shaped by the environment in which our genes, our brains, and our minds ordinarily develop. This is the background against which our particular genetic blueprint was selected during evolution. Many of our remarkable mental and behavioral characteristics do not unfold automatically but need to be nurtured through specific types of stimulation and experience. Our behavioral genes specify capabilities that can remain dormant if they are never activated through experience—in ways that we still do not know enough about. Children need to be spoken to in order to develop language, held in order to develop muscle tone, and loved in order to develop lasting social attachments. They also need to be raised in a nurturing and hospitable environment if they are to grow up to be happy and self-supporting adults—in the same way that seeds need a favorable combination of soil, sunlight, and water to blossom into flowers, even though they contain all the necessary genetic information to do so. The *capacity* to be an upstanding citizen or a social misfit is probably included within the genetic endowment of each of us, but our upbringing and our circumstances tend to shape which it will be. *What* we learn and understand is determined by our experience, but *the way* we learn and the limits of what we can understand are determined by our genes. We are, however, not infinitely adaptable to changes in our environment, as is only too evident from our reactions to the many stresses the modern technological world imposes on us.

Since all behavior has both genetic and learned components that interact to determine what we eventually become, there is little point in arguing about whether nature or nurture is the more important, for both are essential. Our quest should be to identify critical formative influences and discover how they interact to fashion how our brains and behavior develop. We need to know, for example, the crucial types and amounts of experience that growing children require to develop into well-adjusted members of society who are able to interact productively with each other. Although everyone agrees they need an interested, involved, and interacting parent figure to achieve their full potential, no one knows the amount and type of involvement, interest, and interaction that is required—or how this can best be provided by a working single parent, a teenager, or a day-care center. We also know that behavioral growth and maturation are adversely affected by neglect and indifference, as well as by physical, emotional, and sexual abuse; but we do not know enough about the amount, context, and timing of traumatic experiences that irreversibly damage the growing child, or of possible remedies and antidotes that might be able to ameliorate their effects.

OUR BEHAVIORAL REPERTOIRE

Our behavior is the most obvious aspect of our unique heritage and our greatest adaptive advantage in terms of natural selection. Our fine motor skills and coordination, our language and communication, and our incredible array of tools set us apart from all the other species. The most distinctive feature of our behavior, however, is that we respond to what we make of our circumstances, not just to the circumstances themselves. We infer meaning based on our prior experience in ways that no other animal is able to do—which is why there is so much variability in how we respond to a given set of events. Our sense perceptions are even shaped in part by our prevailing conceptions, for we tend to see what we believe we should see, mostly without being aware that we have such biases, although we notice them in others. We construe the meaning of things by fitting them against the mental models we have previously developed, and then respond accordingly.

Scientific concepts of human behavior have largely been built on understanding its more measurable aspects, an approach that has left little room for subjective phenomena such as thinking, feeling, and hoping. One of the great debates about human behavior has been whether what we do is determined by past events and circumstances or by anticipated consequences. Freud, for instance, believed that our behavior is largely determined by our early development and life history, while Skinner argued that it is shaped instead by whether it is rewarded or punished. They were both right as it turns out—at least to some extent. It is not, however, the *actual* consequences that shape our actions in real life but the *expected* ones, for the former are known only in prearranged situations like Skinner's experimental boxes. Our expectations are based, however, on our past experiences and the concepts we have extracted from them, for these form the basis of the models we use to anticipate the outcomes of our actions.[4]

Our brain is the only part of our body that clearly differentiates us from other species, for the structure and function of our other organs are virtually indistinguishable from those of other mammals. Although human brains have a great many similarities with those of other primates, some cortical areas are markedly different, and it seems reasonable to look to these for clues to our uniqueness as a species. The prefrontal cortex is one such area, for it is significantly larger and more developed in humans than in monkeys and apes (Preuss, 2000). Located just behind the forehead, where it constitutes almost one third of the neocortex, it is the reason our foreheads bulge out rather than slant backwards like those of our early ancestors and primate cousins. The prefrontal cortex is one of the last parts of the brain to fully develop, which also points to its more recent evolutionary origin. According to Fuster (1985), the myelin sheaths in this part of the brain are not complete until about two to three years of age, possibly explaining why language, object constancy, and time appreciation do not begin to mature until then. Other parts of this area's neuronal connectivity continue to develop throughout childhood and adolescence, essentially paralleling the growth of our intellectual and reasoning capacities during these years.[5]

Struss and Benson (1986) contend that the prefrontal cortex is responsible for much that is unique about our thinking, language, and behavior. The area plays a central role in the *temporal organization* of thought and behavior, including orchestrating the time sequences involved in language and logical reasoning. It is directly involved in the execution of sequences of behavior that are directed towards future goals that exist in an individual's mind, rather than the external environment. The prefrontal cortex is also responsible for coordinating a number of *executive functions* that utilize prior knowledge and prospective planning in making choices between different courses of action. This process involves analyzing situations, considering alternative behavioral scenarios, selecting the one that seems most advantageous, and inhibiting competing responses and distractions in order to pursue it. The prefrontal cortex is thus the part of the brain that organizes our ability to plan, rehearse, and act on our self-generated ideas about the future.[6]

Ingvar (1985) observes that "the prefrontal cortex handles the temporal organization of behavior and cognition, as well as the action plans for future behavior and cognition which, as they can be retained and recalled, can be termed *memories of the future*. It is suggested that these form the basis for anticipation and expectation, as well as for the short- and long-term planning of a goal-directed behavioral and cognitive repertoire." He also indicates that "experimental and clinical observation strongly support the idea that the prefrontal cortex is selectively responsible for the temporal structuring of future behavior and cognition due to its seemingly specific capacity to handle serial information and to extract causal relations from such information." As Fuster (1997) observes, the prefrontal cortex appears to be well-suited for coordinating sensory input, stored information, "off-line" processing, and then initiating action, since it has a great profusion of reciprocal connections with all of the cortical and subcortical areas implicated in information processing, emotional regulation, and behavioral response. Arnsten (1998) remarks: "The prefrontal cortex recalls memories from long-term storage and uses these representations to effectively guide behavior, freeing us from responding only to our immediate environment, inhibiting inappropriate responses or distractions, and allowing us to plan and organize."

Patients with prefrontal damage are generally unable to initiate and carry out goal-directed behavior that is associated with deliberation and choice, even though they may have no trouble executing old, well-rehearsed routines. Brain lesions in this area give rise to states that are characterized by what has been called a *loss of the future*, typically involving a lack of initiative and an inability to foresee the consequences of one's own behavior. Affected individuals tend to live in the present without any idea of what is likely to happen later on, existing without ambition, foresight, or spontaneity. Bechra et al. (1994) report that, despite otherwise normal intellectual functions, prefrontally damaged patients are "oblivious to the future consequences of their actions, and seem to be guided by immediate prospects only." Apathy is thus a commonly encountered symptom among these individuals; they show little interest in anything other than meeting their immediate needs. They may act impulsively, show poor emotional control, and engage in foolhardy actions, because they are unable to inhibit their responses and lack the foresight needed to worry about what might befall them. Individuals with significantly impaired prefrontal function generally face each day without any hope that things will get better, but also without any fear of their getting worse. As Ingvar (1985) notes, prefrontal brain damage disrupts our ability to plan, rehearse, and then act on ideas of future action.[7]

Anderson et al. (1999) report that adults who experienced substantial damage to the prefrontal cortex while they were young children seem predisposed to grow up with little regard for social conventions or the welfare of others, despite having intact cognitive skills. They resemble individuals with a sociopathic personality disorder, for they seem to show the same type of irresponsibility, disregard for moral standards, and lack of remorse for what they do. Patients whose prefrontal lesions develop when they are adults do not show the same sort of antisocial behavior. This raises the possibility that antisocial individuals may have an incompletely developed prefrontal cortex, possibly because stresses experienced during early childhood interfered with the development of a functional system for representing the world—with the result that they are unable to foresee the consequences of their actions. Recent studies of men with antisocial personality disorder and of certain violent offenders have, in fact, reported significantly reduced prefrontal functioning. Stoddard et al. (1996) and Raine et al. (1997) report reduced activity of the prefrontal cortex in a group of forty-one men incarcerated for murder. Raine et al. (2000) found an average 11 percent reduction in the volume of neuronal gray matter in the prefrontal cortex in a group of twenty-one individuals with antisocial personality disorder, as compared to controls. Deckel et al. (1996) found that antisocial personality disorder was associated with decreased frontal lobe function as measured by electro-encephalographic and neuropsychological testing. It thus seems possible that the ability to plan future actions may be compromised by traumatic experiences during childhood that interfere with the full development of this part of the brain.[8]

MALFUNCTIONS OF THE MIND

Mental illnesses are distinctly human illnesses, part of the price we pay for having such unique brains. Other species can be afflicted with diabetes, cancer, heart disease, and so on, but they do not suffer from depression, panic disorder, or schizophrenia in the way we do. Mental illnesses represent malfunctions of the distinctly human aspects of our brains, such as thinking, remembering, imagining, and anticipating. In many ways, they are also disorders of human consciousness, for the emotional suffering that characterizes them would be greatly reduced if we were not consciously aware of our past experience and anticipated future. Although higher animals can show disturbed, inappropriate, and maladaptive behaviors in response to overwhelming stress or experimental intervention, these responses are not true replicas of human disorders, even though some of the resultant symptoms resemble those found in mental illnesses. In fact, our understanding of human mental disorders has lagged behind our understanding of our physical ones largely because there are no naturally occurring animal models that can be used to investigate and understand these conditions. Ironically, although mentally ill individuals have often been stigmatized and at times been considered to be less than fully human, their illnesses actually affirm their humanity.[9]

Mental illnesses are often referred to as *emotional illnesses* because they are accompanied by intense or inappropriate emotion. The emotional system is generally not disordered in these individuals, however, but is usually working overtime to keep up with their perceptions of the world—for the emotions that people with mental illnesses endure are generally appropriate to how they experience and interpret what they encounter. Rather, it is the representational systems they have developed to understand and give meaning to the world that appear to be disordered. Thus, while the emotional turmoil that accompanies mental illnesses may not make sense to the outside observer, it is generally in keeping with the individual's own beliefs and ideas. Helping emotionally troubled individuals focus their attention on the immediate present will usually relieve some of their distress, since it provides a temporary respite from the worries about the past and concerns with the future that plague them. People who live entirely in the present generally do not experience the types of suffering or impairment that characterize mental illnesses, even though they may become nervous, unhappy, or apathetic in response to their current circumstances.

Mental illnesses offer a window for examining normal mental functioning, in much the same way that physical illnesses provide an opportunity for understanding how the healthy body operates. We first gained an inkling about the brain's intricate chemical messenger systems in the 1960s, for instance, from studying how the drugs that relieve these disorders work. Since then, scientists have begun to piece together a general understanding of the neural mechanisms on which both normal and abnormal mental function are built. Modern imaging techniques now make it possible to study the brain's chemical systems in both affected and unaffected individuals as they think about various topics, experience different emotions, and perform given tasks. It appears from these studies that mental illness and mental health are made from the same cloth—for no brain substances have yet been found that are unique to these disorders. We thus have a pressing need to understand mental illnesses better, not just for the sake of helping those who are affected, but because of the crucial insights they can provide about how our brains and minds ordinarily go about determining our thoughts, our feelings, and our behavior.[10]

One of the major challenges facing humankind today is to better under-stand the factors that shape and determine human behavior—so that we can begin to address the problems that threaten our desired way of life. We need to know enough about our own nature and its limits to be able to work out how we should raise and educate our children, stay healthy, get along with each other, enjoy our gifts, and govern ourselves effectively. We live out our lives today in complex social and economic environments that we have created but neither fully understand nor fully control. Despite all of our material successes, we are not as confident about the idea of progress as we once were, for we are faced with mounting concerns about the sustainability of our environment and way of life. We are surrounded with signs of stress and social disruption—unhappiness, anxiety, cynicism, di-vorce, suicide, violence, drug abuse, and family break-down.

Brand (1999) observes: "Civilization is revving itself into a patholog-ically short attention span. The trend might be coming from the accelera-tion of technology, the short-horizon perspective of market-driven econo-mies, the next-election perspectives of democracies, or the distractions of personal multitasking. All are on the increase. Some sort of balancing corrective to the short-sightedness is needed—some mechanism or myth that encourages the long view and the taking of long-term responsibility." Garbarino (1988) also stresses that we need to be concerned about the future, to act in ways that preserve the environment, and to try to alleviate human inequities if we want to leave a world worth living in for succeeding generations. But it is difficult enough going without something in order to enhance our *own* future well-being, let alone doing it to benefit unknown generations that have yet to come. It is also hard to make sacrifices for future threats that are not yet certain, even when we know that by the time they become certain it may be too late to do anything about them.[11]

Our incredible journey over the last ten thousand years has been fueled by an ever-increasing accumulation of knowledge about the uni-verse in which we live. We now need to turn our energies to understanding the unique ways in which we, ourselves, get molded and function, so that we can live in greater harmony with each other and with the world around us—and raise our children so that they will be able to do the same. The human mind and the human brain are among the last great frontiers of science, complex and challenging entities that contain the very essence of our humanity. We need to use them to figure out how they determine what we do—to understand ourselves as we actually are, rather than in terms of the ideologies and superstitions we have been raised to believe. As Salk (1972) observes, "the mind does not reveal itself to itself except indirectly. The mind must surmise what the mind is, what its elements are, and how it works. The individual mind needs to become conscious enough of its own nature, of its own workings, to be able to increase conscious control that will permit the making of judgments based upon values derived from nature." The hope is not to change human nature but to understand it sufficiently to be able to shape our social, economic, and political environments so that they bring out the best in us, not the worst.

We are without doubt the most remarkable of nature's creatures, but we are creatures none the less, bound by all of the natural world's rules and obligations. We are as much a part of the ecological landscape as every other living being, and our survival is no more guaranteed than theirs. We need to stop acting as if we were immune to the laws of nature and as if the world were endlessly indestructible, ours to do with as we please. If we want to safeguard the legacy that has been passed on to us and ensure that there will be a future that our heirs can enjoy, we must discover how to refrain from polluting our minds with prejudice, our brains with drugs, our society with violence, and our environment with toxic substances. We need to recognize more clearly the price we pay for being out of tune with our surroundings and with each other. As Farb (1978) observes, "humankind is apparently the first species on the planet that has ever been threatened by its own biological success."[12]

Our ability to predict the future is a two-edged sword. If we can see good times ahead as we peer into the crystal ball, we generate hope and energy; but if what we see is dark and foreboding, we become weighed down with inaction and despair. Both reactions are, to some extent, self-fulfilling, for what we come to believe shapes how we respond to it. Hope gives us only possibilities, not guarantees; but it mobilizes us to act, to analyze and understand our problems, and to try to solve them. Realistic hopes are, unfortunately, difficult to come by in times of crisis and uncertainty. However, we will never know whether we are able to give up our short-sighted, destructive ways, forgive age-old rivalries, and work together for the common good if we do not try—or do not believe we have the talent and ingenuity needed to tackle these problems. Medawar (1972) contends: "To deride the hope of progress is the ultimate fatuity, the last word in poverty of spirit and meanness of mind. There is no need to be dismayed by the fact that we cannot yet envisage a definitive solution of our problems, a resting place beyond which we need not try to go." He sides with Francis Bacon (1561–1626), who remarked, "The greatest obstacle to the growth of understanding is that men despair and think things impossible." In Greek mythology, when Prometheus's brother ignored a warning not to accept any gifts from the gods and took Pandora as his bride, she brought with her a box containing every human ill. When he opened Pandora's box, all the evil escaped into the world. All that was left in the box was *hope*.

Notes

1. Rycroft (1979) quotes John Cohen: "But although life without hope is unthinkable, psychology without hope is not, judging by the conspicuous absence of any study of hope in the literature." There have, however, been at least two attempts to formulate a psychology of hope. Stotland (1969) outlines a cognitive model that defines hope as an expectation of attaining a goal, either in the present or in the future. He also applies the concept to experimental animals pushing a lever in the *hope* of getting a reward, rather than viewing hope as an experience that is independent of current environmental stimuli. Snyder (1994 & 2000) also offers a cognitive model that views hope as a specific way of thinking about oneself that is derived from a combination of willpower and what he calls *waypower*, by which he means having a pathway towards a goal that one wants to achieve. He has developed scales that measure hope by assessing willpower and waypower from responses to questionnaires and finds it correlated with achievement and success.

2. A variety of historical individuals have commented on hope. Aristotle (384–322 BC) observed that "hope was a waking dream"; Terence (195–159 BC) maintained that "where there's life, there's hope"; Martin Luther (1483–1546) said, "Everything that is done in the world is done for hope"; Shakespeare (1564–1616) wrote, "The miserable have no other medicine, but only hope"; Alexander Pope (1688–1744) held that "hope springs eternal in the human breast"; Samuel Johnson (1709–1784) thought that hope was "perhaps the chief happiness which this world affords"; Victor Hugo (1802–1885) declared that hope was "the word that God has written on the brow of every man"; Erich Fromm (1900–1980) remarked that "to hope is an essential condition of being human, if man gives up all hope, he has left behind his own humanity"; and Norman Cousins (1915–1990) believed that "the capacity for hope is the most significant fact in life; it provides human beings with a sense of destination and the energy to get started." Not all comments have been favorable, however. Many ancient Greeks were fatalists who, believing that everything was predetermined and unchangeable, thought that

hope was a dangerous illusion. Shelley (1792–1822), a Romantic, observed that "worse than despair, worse than the bitterness of death, is hope"; and Nietzsche (1844–1900) declared, "Hope is the worst of all evils, for it prolongs the torment of man."

3. Thomas Aquinas (1267) defines hope as "the movement of appetite aroused by the perception of what is agreeable, future, arduous and possible of attainment." Other definitions include: "an expectation greater than zero of achieving a goal" (Stotland, 1969) and "an arduous search for a future good of some kind that is realistically possible, but not yet visible" (Lynch, 1974). Shackle (1990) points out that "hopes differ from fantasies in that they involve imaginative expectations that are constrained by what we believe may plausibly happen. Enjoyment by anticipation is not derived from mere day dreams, but by imagining a future course of events which seems credible to us as an outcome of our planned actions."

4. Haith et al. (1994) observe, "In light of the importance of future-orientation in organisms, it is puzzling that so little attention has been paid to future-oriented processes in the psychological literature." They believe that part of the reason is that psychology has focused so heavily on how organisms respond to measurable environmental stimuli. Gell (1992) mentions the French language distinction, and Lynch (1974) quotes St. Paul (Romans 8:24, KJV).

5. Zimbardo (1994) believes that "there is no psychological variable or process that exerts a greater influence across a wider range of human thoughts, feelings, and actions than does psychological time orientation." According to Samuel Johnson: "The future is purchased by the present. It is not possible to secure distant or permanent happiness but by the forbearance of some immediate gratification" (Brand, 1999). The Dalai Lama and Cutler (1998) also point out: "Dealing with expectations is a tricky issue. If you have excessive expectations without a proper foundation, that usually leads to problems; on the other hand, without expectation and hope, there can be no progress. Some hope is essential, but finding the proper balance is not easy."

6. Byrne (1995) reviews the ability of other species to anticipate the future. His conclusion is that "all these signs of forethought concern items relevant to the animals' current motivational state, their current goal. Humans plan beyond their current needs and desires."

7. Faith, hope, and charity are the three heavenly graces of Christian theology, where God is both the source and the end of hope. The future these religious hopes are concerned with is generally not of this world, however, but of heaven and a perpetual afterlife (Rycroft, 1979).

8. Awbrey (1999) claims, along with Kierkegaard, that melancholy is a spiritual sickness caused by humanity's alienation from God, not just a mental or emotional disorder. While this may be true for some individuals, it is not for most.

9. Seligman (1991) and Chang (2001) review studies of the effects of optimism and pessimism. Seligman (2002) proposes that people can maximize their potential for fulfillment by focusing on positive emotions. Cousins (1989) and Tiger (1979) discuss the biological effects of hope and optimism. They provide anecdotal support for their belief that positive emotions can influence the outcome of illness through their impact

on the immune system. Most people find it easier to accept the idea that emotions affect a patient's subjective symptoms of *illness*, rather than a physician's objective findings of *disease* (Reading, 1977).

10. White, Tursky and Schwartz (1985) review studies of the placebo response, while Beecher (1995) describes the cardiac pain one. Price and Barrell (1999) explore the role of expectation in the placebo relief of pain.

11. Frank (1961) points out that the effectiveness of medical care in less developed countries (and in more developed ones until recent times) depended on the mobilization of positive expectancies by the shaman or physician, based on the special authority sick individuals invested in them. Menninger believed that it is part of the physician's job to "keep alive the little candle of hope, so that it does not weaken, sputter and go out" (1959).

12. Garber and Seligman (1980) review studies of human helplessness. Seligman (1975) notes that helplessness is associated with a cognitive appraisal style in which individuals overly interpret events in a pessimistic way, and that this can be modified through cognitive training. He claims that people who get depressed can be treated by teaching them to become more optimistic.

13. Fear and anxiety can also be triggered by uncertainties about *current* environmental events, not just future ones, which is why they occur in human infants, present-oriented individuals, and other species.

CHAPTER 2. PREDICTING THE FUTURE

1. Dennett (1991) maintains that the fundamental purpose of the brain is to produce a future—that our brains are, in essence, *anticipation machines*. Other animals are only capable of what he calls *proximal anticipation*, behavior that is appropriate to what is in their immediate future. He notes that humans build a mental model of the world, based on information they have gleaned from experience, and use this to generate rules and principles that enable them to make predictions that are independent of what is going on in their current environment. Craik (1943) was probably the first to conceive of the brain as a prediction machine. He proposed that much of our thinking involved the mental simulation of possible future outcomes.

2. Machiavelli (1520) comments: "Whoever wishes to foresee the future must consult the past: for human events ever resemble those of previous times. This arises from the fact that they are produced by men who ever have been, and ever will be, animated by the same passions, and thus they necessarily have the same result." Schumacher (1973) notes: "All men at all times have been wanting to know the future. The ancient Chinese used to consult the *I Ching* which is reputed to be the oldest book of mankind. It is based on the conviction that, while everything changes all the time, change itself is unchanging and conforms to certain ascertainable metaphysical laws."

3. Frank (1961) observes: "For it is only to the extent that a person can successfully predict the results of his acts that he can behave in such a way as to maximize his chances for success and minimize those for failure. Thus everyone is strongly motivated constantly to check the validity of his assumptions, and every act is both a

consequence of a more or less explicit expectation and a test of its validity. If the consequences of the act fail to confirm the prediction, the person is in trouble. He must either modify his expectations and the corresponding behavior or resort to maneuvers to conceal their incorrectness and evade their unfortunate consequences." Wright (1984) notes that many of us also act in ways that gather additional information, which we use to revise our initial predictions in a Baynesian-like manner to make them more accurate; such behaviors include sending up a trial balloon, probing for an initial response, or discussing the options with friends.

4. Kahneman and Tversky (2000) explore the impact that subjective factors have on the utility and value considerations used in decision making.

5. Stewart (2000) observes that "actions that are based on predictions lead to two types of errors. One is when an event that is predicted does not occur (i.e., a false alarm); the other is when an event occurs but is not predicted (i.e., a surprise). There is an inevitable trade-off between these two kinds of errors, since steps taken to reduce one unavoidably increase the other."

6. Burke (2000) outlines the effect that the growth of knowledge has had on Western societies over the past four centuries, including the impact of the printing press, libraries, scientific research, and universities.

7. The model has a number of similarities to the stages of future-oriented behavior proposed by Norman (1988): "(a) forming the goal and deciding on the desired outcome, (b) forming the intention and deciding to do something to achieve the goal, (c) specifying the action or action sequence and formulating a plan to do it, (d) executing the action or actions, (e) perceiving the state of the world and the effects of the action, (f) interpreting the state of the world, and (g) evaluating the outcome in respect to the initial goal."

8. Shackle (1962) observes: "We decide on one particular course of action out of a number of rival courses because this one gives us, as an immediately present experience, the most enjoyment by *anticipation* of its outcome." He points out: "The real incentive for embarking on some given venture, whose objective results will not develop and their character become known until some date in the future, is the *immediate* mental experience which the decision to embark on this course will give us, namely, the *enjoyment by anticipation* of a high level of success."

9. Maddux (1999) notes that the expectancy construct and various expectancy and expectancy-value theories are among the most thoroughly investigated models in psychology. Feather (1982) outlines how expectation-value models differ from simple stimulus-response paradigms of behavior by emphasizing the role of cognitive functions in initiating behavior and responding to environmental information. Goldman (2002) outlines how expectancy theories can be used to understand why people use and abuse alcohol and drugs.

10. McHugh and Slavney (1998) distinguish between biologically determined motivations (e.g., for food and sex) and socially determined ones (e.g., for wealth and prestige).

11. Trefil (1997) notes that "it might turn out that when you put a sufficiently

complex system together, you will be unable to predict what its properties are in practice because the connection between the individual parts and the final behavior is too complicated to know." Sarewitz, Pielke and Byerly (2000) also point out that "the theoretical and technical difficulties of predicting complex natural systems are immense, and the magnitude of the uncertainties associated with such predictions may be not only large, but also themselves highly uncertain." Merry (1995) concurs: "Uncertainty, impredictability, complexity, and chaos are . . . natural, legitimate, necessary, inescapable aspects of reality and will never go away. Complex systems abound in the real world, and they reflect the world's inherent irregularity."

12. Brunner (2000) notes that "the potential to predict human behavior with precision, scope and accuracy is *limited* because human behavior is not determined by fundamental laws. Instead, human behavior stems most directly from choices and decisions that are contingent upon individual, unavoidably subjective perspectives, or internal models." Shackle (1990) points out that our sense of free will is, however, derived from our ignorance of the future, for as we can only conjecture about the consequences of our actions, we make different choices depending on how we see them. Schumacher (1973) claims that life is only worth living because it is sufficiently unpredictable to make it interesting.

13. Franklin (2001) notes that certain events are too complex for us to be able to understand all of the determining (causal) factors, so we call them accidents or chance events.

14. Shackle (1962) believed that the statistical theories of probability, which are based on the outcomes of indefinitely repeated trials, are not the way we actually deal with the everyday uncertainties that face us, for actuarial principles tell us nothing about what will happen in a particular instance. He uses the concept of surprise as a way of estimating this type of probability by ascertaining how surprised individuals would be if their hoped-for futures did not eventuate. The more certain we are that an event will happen, the more surprised we will be if it does not.

CHAPTER 3. THE INTERNAL REPRESENTATION OF
THE EXTERNAL WORLD

1. As Johnston (1999) points out, "few of us realize that our brain creates what is, in effect, a virtual reality. The idea is so contrary to our common sense that few rational people would consider such a proposal to be an important scientific insight that is essential for understanding human nature, but it is." Mountcastle (1975) also observes: "Each of us believes himself to live directly within the world that surrounds him, to sense its objects and events precisely, to live in real and current time. These are perceptual illusions, for each of us confronts the world from a brain linked to what is 'out there' by a few million fragile sensory nerve fibres. These are our only information channels, our lifelines to reality. These sensory nerve fibres are not high-fidelity recorders, for they accentuate certain stimulus features, neglect other. The central neuron is a story-teller with regard to the afferent nerve fibres; and he is never completely trustworthy, allowing distortions of quality and measure, within a strained but

isomorphic spatial relation between 'outside' and 'inside.' Sensation is an abstraction, not a replication of the real world."

2. Gopnik and Melzoff (1996), Perner (1991) and Rogers, Rutherford, and Bibby (1992) discuss the nature of mental representations.

3. Bickerton (1995) uses the terms *primary representation* and *secondary representation* to refer to sensory and symbolic representations. Primary representations portray specific entities (e.g., *Fido, my home*), while secondary ones stand for abstract concepts and categories (e.g., *dog, house*) that are based on words and ideas, although not necessarily words as we know them. He notes that secondary representations also involve some form of syntax that denotes whether an imagined entity is in the past, the present, or the future, or whether it is a particular or general instance—as they are not limited by the tangible restrictions that characterize primary representations.

4. Vauclair (1996) reviews the evidence for representation in birds and mammals. As an example of spatial representation, he describes how Clark's Nutcrackers harvest pine seeds during the late summer and hide them in thousands of discrete subterranean caches which they are apparently able to locate when they subsequently need them. He notes, however, that human language is a symbolic representational system that enables us to refer to objects or events that are remote in time and place and to think about things that may never occur, while the communication systems of other animals are limited to conveying information about the present.

5. Gopnik and Melzoff (1996) believe that infants develop theories, which they test against further experience, just like scientists, using further input to confirm or disconfirm already-formed beliefs.

6. Craik (1943) defines a model as "any physical or chemical system which has a similar relation-structure to that of the process it imitates," and maintains that "if an organism carries a 'small-scale model' of external reality and of its own possible actions within its head, it is able to try out various alternatives, conclude which is the best of them, react to future situations before they arise, utilize the knowledge of past events in dealing with the present and the future, and in every way to react in a much fuller, safer, and more competent manner to the emergencies which face it." Rivett (1972) notes that "the history of man is a history of model building, a constant search for pattern and for generalization." He points out that "a model is first of all a convenient way of representing the total experience we possess, of then deducing from that experience whether we are in the presence of pattern and law and, if so, of showing how such patterns and laws can be used to predict the future."

7. Suppe (1977) notes that psychology did not become a separate discipline from philosophy until the introduction of experimentation in the late nineteenth century, and that epistemology, the branch of philosophy that deals with the nature of knowledge, parallels the psychological understanding of how we know and understand the world, although from a different perspective.

8. Gigerenzer and Murray (1987) discuss how the brain uses past experience to estimate the future consequences of the actions contemplated during the process of

rational decision making. Dawes (1988) believes that "rational decisions are based on an assessment of future possibilities and probabilities; the past is relevant only insofar as it provides information about possible and probable futures." Calvin (1996) quotes John Holland (*Daedalus*, Winter, 1992): "An internal model allows a system to look ahead to the future consequences of current actions, without actually committing itself to those actions. In particular, the system can avoid acts that would set it irretrievably down some road to future disaster."

9. Kelly's theory of personal constructs is one of the forerunners of modern cognitive psychology. He proposes that every construct includes an opposite that helps define it: *up* and *down*, *heavy* and *light*, *chair* and *non-chair*. *Beauty* and *ugliness* are thus part of the same construct in this system, with each depending on the other for its meaning. Fauconnier and Turner (2002) believe it is the *blending* of such concepts that most distinguishes human cognition.

10. The terms *structural* and *functional* are used here to refer to the variety of noncasual relationships that link various objects and events in our minds. They imply that there is some form of connection between the neuronal representations of the related entities, so that activating a memory or thought of one tends to activate the representation of the other. Hundert (1989) notes that Hume (1711–1776) proposed six different types of noncausal relationships: resemblance, identity, relations of time and place, proportion in quantity or number, degrees in any quality, and contrariety. Other noncausal relationships include: associative (*blonde* and *hair*), conceptual (*radius* and *diameter*), utilitarian (*gasoline* and *automobile*), and correlation (*cigarette smoking* and *lung cancer*). Hundert credits Kant (1724–1804) with being the first modern philosopher to point out that relationships between entities in the environment cannot be directly experienced, only inferred.

11. Eugen Bleuler, who first introduced the term *schizophrenia*, believed that *loose associations* were the hallmark of the thought disorder that characterizes this illness. The fact that the associations made by these individuals have little apparent logical connection to each other indicates that their brains may not connect related entities in the same way that the nonschizophrenic ones do and may explain the difficulty these individuals have in understanding abstractions.

12. Delbanco (1999) believes that people organize their sensations and experiences into a plausible story that helps them navigate through life. He notes that when an individual's personal story leads somewhere, it gives them hope. He regards culture as a sustained narrative that is shared by a number of people and gives meaning to the world in which they live.

13. Yalom (1980) observes that people who believe that their life has no meaning tend to feel lost and alienated. He reviews the effect that existential concerns about death, freedom, isolation, and meaninglessness have on our sense of mental well-being.

14. Skinner (1972) does not agree with the concept of an autonomous self. He believes that "a scientific analysis of behavior dispossesses man and turns the control he is said to have exerted over to the environment. The individual is controlled by the

world around him, and in large part by other men. A person does not act upon the world, the world acts upon him." This behavioristic view assumes that individuals are only passive responders, not active inteveners who help shape their own destinies.

15. The idea that we are only capable of understanding something in relation to something else is consistent with Einstein's notions of relativity and Heisenberg's observation that it is not possible to determine both the position and the momentum of a subatomic particle, such as an electron, because one has to be held constant in order to measure the other. It is also compatible with Gödel's theorem that there are propositions that can be neither proven nor disproven within any given mathematical system (Trefil 1997).

16. Theories are explanatory models that try to explicate the relationships between different aspects of the natural world, abstract principles that bind a series of facts together. Hypotheses, on the other hand, are testable propositions that are derived from them. A theory is not necessarily invalidated when a particular hypothesis is found to be untrue, but it becomes increasingly suspect if a number of hypotheses turn out to be wrong. Conversely, while validating a given hypothesis does not prove the theory behind it, validating several of them makes the theory more likely to be true. Popper (1935) believed, however, that although the system that the brain uses to process information is like the scientific method, it is not identical to it, because it is based on induction—generalizing from a particular observation and making predictions on this basis—rather than deduction.

17. Horney (1939) observes that "the system of theories which Freud has gradually developed is so consistent that when one is entrenched in them it is difficult to make observations unbiased by his way of thinking."

CHAPTER 4. THE PROCESSING OF INFORMATION

1. Descartes's separation of mind and body was an attempt to explain the differences between the mental properties of humans and those of other animals. His ideas about the workings of the body were influenced by the successes that mechanical explanations had proved in understanding the workings of the physical universe. Galileo had asserted a few years earlier that science should only be concerned with things that could be weighed and measured and should ignore mental qualities, like meaning and value.

2. Discussion of the human mind can be found in Broadwell (1994), Edelman (1992), Humphrey (1992), Jackendoff (1994), and Pinker (1997). Russell (1921), Ryle (1949), and Searle (1992) offer philosophical perspectives on the relation between mind and brain. Introductions to the human brain can be found in Allman (1999), LeDoux (2002), Restak (1994), Restak (1995), Squire (1987), and Wade (1998). Calvin (1996) and Damasio (1994) provide more technical overviews, and Jastrow (1981) depicts the evolution of the human brain for nonspecialists. Gazzaniga (1998) presents a case for mental processes' being mostly shaped by genes, rather than experience. Kandel, Schwartz and Jessell (2000) provide a comprehensive review of neuroscience for the more advanced reader.

3. The number of neurons in the human cerebral cortex is about the same as the number of stars in our galaxy. Counting at the rate of one per second, it would take more than three thousand years to count all of their synaptic connections. That no one seems ever to have lost weight by thinking too much seems to indicate that consciousness comprises only a small part of the brain's metabolic activity.

4. Gregory (1986) observes that "computers cannot understand symbols (or indeed anything else either), though they can manipulate symbols according to formal rules with consummate speed and accuracy, far surpassing our own fumbling efforts. They do not understand the questions they are asked or the answers they provide." Trefil (1997) argues that brains and computers are not really all that alike, that they work in different ways and are good at different things. Dreyfus (1979) maintains that building a computer that can function like the human brain and achieve consciousness is a practical impossibility, despite its popularity in science fiction stories.

5. Spradlin and Porterfield (1979) observe that the division of human information processing into two distinct components was proposed by a number of individuals over the years, including Freud (primary and secondary process), Pavlov (first and second signaling systems), Pribram (digital and analogical systems), and Young (abstract and maplike systems). They believe that these formulations all contain the same essential division into: (a) an analog system in which data is integrated continuously into maplike pictures or gestalts, and (b) a digital system in which data are processed into individual units or segments that can be combined to form new information patterns. They point out that the latter enables us to plot our perceptions in a logical sequence on a space-time grid, which is what allows us to predict future data. Norwich (1993) notes that analog systems transmit information about continuous phenomena, while digital ones involve discrete data (e.g., on/off). Continuous variables can be converted into digital ones, however, as in digitizing a photograph image or television transmission.

6. Johnson (1992) describes research about the neural basis of learning.

7. Edelman and Tononi (2000) note that "the pervasive automatization in our adult lives suggests that conscious control is exerted only at critical junctures, when a definite choice or a plan has to be made."

8. Our brains are specially endowed with the capacity to recognize human faces, so that a familiar face can be recognized from almost any angle in less than 250 milliseconds. Rather than separately storing each face we have ever seen, with the expression, angle, distance, and light of each time we have seen it, it seems likely that we store faces in some kind of generic form, and then encode only how such prototypes have to be modified to represent particular individuals at particular times. Churchland (1996) describes how a coding system based on deviations from a prototypic representation would make this possible.

9. Nonhuman primates and some other higher mammals are able to process simple forms of symbolic information, in much the same way that humans process the meaning of nonverbal signs and signals. While our ability to understand the meaning of a smile, a scream, or a grimace is innate, we learn the meaning of other nonverbal signals through associations, as with stop signs, patriotic flags, or trademarks. Language is,

however, more than a series of isolated symbols. It is an elaborate *system* of symbols in which the sounds and images of its component elements are arranged in specified ways that convey information. Language is discussed further in Chapter 9.

10. McDougall (1921) observes that "we are *confident* if we assume blithely that desire will be realized, *hopeful* if we anticipate that it will be realized but appreciate the contingencies that could arise to prevent this, *despondent* if we think it unlikely to be realized, *disappointed* if we lose all expectation of it being realized while still continuing to desire it, and *despair* if we come to believe that it will never be realized."

11. The observations about rotten eggs and sugar are from Johnston (1999). The nature of emotion is discussed further in Chapter 7.

12. The two sides of the cerebral cortex tend to process different aspects of the information our sensory system receives, with objects and events generally being perceived as wholes by the right hemisphere and as component parts by the left one. The right hemisphere is thus usually dominant for nonverbal, pattern-recognition, and spatial tasks, such as reading maps, copying designs, interpreting facial expressions, and appreciating music. The left hemisphere is usually dominant for speech and language, as well as for temporal sequencing and calculation. As Hellige (1993) points out, the purpose these hemispheric differences serve or how they arose during evolution is not clear. Details of how neural systems process information can be found in Calvin (1996), Crick (1994), Edelman (1992), Jackendoff (1994), Restak (1994), Squire (1987), and Trehub (1991).

13. Panksepp (1998) provides a comprehensive review of the neurobiology of emotion.

14. Damasio (1994) notes: "Images are not stored as facsimile pictures of things, events, words, or sentences. The brain does not file Polaroid pictures of people, objects, landscapes, nor audiotapes of music and speech. There seem to be no permanently stored pictures of anything, even miniaturized microfiches. Whenever we recall a given object or face or scene, we do not get an exact reproduction, but rather an interpretation, a newly reconstructed version of the original."

15. The difference between sensory stimuli and information is evident in a roller-coaster ride, in which there is lots of stimulation but relatively little information. Information depends on a discernible pattern that can be meaningfully differentiated from a random configuration of the same elements. Pullum (1991) believes that the often-quoted anecdote about the ability of Eskimos to distinguish numerous types of snow is a hoax.

16. Tye (1995) outlines how the retina captures the patterns of physical energy that represent visual information and transforms them into corresponding neuronal coding patterns. The brain also converts the sound patterns of the verbal symbols we hear into patterns of neuronal symbols that uniquely represent them, and it does the opposite conversion when we speak. Barrow (1991) points out that the brain is an algorithmic compressor that enables us to abbreviate the information content of our everyday experience by discerning the nonrandom patterns of nature. A nonrandom string of numbers is one which can be represented by an abbreviated string (i.e., it can

be compressed), while a random string is one in which this is not possible—for it contains no discernible order.

17. Although all real systems are open and infinitely interconnected with other systems, we are able to act as if they are closed and independent at times without too great a distortion. Closed systems are surrounded by impermeable boundaries across which no interactions are possible—otherwise they would be open.

CHAPTER 5. THE ROLE OF LEARNING AND MEMORY

1. Learning and memory have generally been viewed as separate processes, largely because of the different ways we access and study them. They have usually been investigated indirectly, by observing changes in *behavior* in response to environmental contingencies, as with Pavlov's dogs and Skinner's pigeons, but current neurobiological studies show promise of discovering their actual mechanisms.

2. All animals modify their behavior as a result of what they experience, for even single-cell organisms habituate. Innate reinforcers like food, sex, and security can become associated with a variety of other experiences that further shape an individual's behavior.

3. Most texts pay little attention to imitative learning, possibly because it does not readily occur in the laboratory animals that are usually studied. Blackmore (1999) believes that imitation is the main way that cultural information is transmitted in humans. Yando, Seitz and Zigler (1978) provide an overview of research on imitative learning.

4. Plotkin (1994) believes that all behavioral adaptations represent a form of knowledge. He defines knowledge as information about the world and about how to adapt to it that is encoded by unique patterns in our genes and our neuronal connections.

5. Rose (1992) observes that we are the only species that has been able to create a world of artificial memory by transcribing our memories onto papyrus, wax tablets, electronic screens, and the like. These make it possible for us to share a "collective memory" about the shared history of our group. The nongenetic transmission of information from generation to generation is discussed further in Chapter 8.

6. Schacter (1996) provides a helpful overview of memory for the general reader. Other sources of information about this topic include: Baars (1997), Broadwell (1994), Brown (1976), Cohen (1996), Foster and Jelicic (1999), Loftus and Loftus (1976), Restak (1994), Rose (1992), Schacter and Tulving (1994), Tulving (2000), and Tulving and Craik (2000). Several systems have been proposed for classifying memory, each a little different from the other. The one used here is consistent with the scheme proposed by Tulving and Donaldson (1972), as well as with the previous discussion of information processing. Recall and recognition are more clearly differentiated in the present approach, where the former is linked to symbolic (semantic) memory and the latter to sensory (episodic) memory. Somatic and emotional memory are not usually included in other classification systems, possibly because they do not lend themselves to the type of research usually used to study memory.

7. Not everyone agrees that recall and recognition are distinct memory processes,

partly because the terms are not always defined the same way. Rose (1992), for instance, defines recall as the expression of modified behavior at some time subsequent to the initial learning, without clearly differentiating it from recognition. Tulving (1976) suggests that part of the difficulty is that the terms are often used to refer to the experimental procedures used to study them, rather than the phenomena themselves. That spontaneous, noncued recall seems to be limited to humans and that sensory memories of smell, touch, taste, and pain can be recognized but not recalled argue strongly for recall's being associated with the symbolic processing system. Roediger, Buckner, and McDermott (1999) review the experimental data that support the theory that recall and recognition are involved in separate memory systems.

8. Hobson (1999) believes that some people are able to recall previously experienced odors, mostly in association with images of the particular entities that are involved.

9. Schank (1982) proposed the concept of *scripts* to explain how we remember the time sequences involved in routine and repetitive events. He defined them as neuronal structures that describe appropriate sequences of events in a particular context.

10. Broadwell (1994) notes a study in which subjects were shown 2,500 different color slides for ten seconds each and ten days later were able to recognize which ones they had previously seen with 90 percent accuracy. Standing (1973) reports a similar study in which subjects were able identify over 10,000 pictures with 66 percent accuracy two days after having been shown each of them for five seconds. In neither case were the subjects able to otherwise recall the items.

11. Dudai (1989), Rose (1992), Squire (1987), and Squire and Kandel (1999) provide introductions to the neurobiology of memory and learning.

12. Tinbergen (1955) reports studies showing that both the feeding responses of gulls and face recognition in human infants are elicited by only a few key features, not the entire presenting images. The same sort of informational parsimony probably characterizes a number of biological systems, so that only the key features of a stimulus are needed to produce the needed response. This may explain why we can recognize a face more easily than we can recall its details—and why there are so few close-ups of people in our dreams and fantasies. Lynn and McConkey (1998) and Loftus (2000) review the variety of distortions that occur in the way recalled memories are reconstructed; some are due to external suggestion, some to the individual's own belief system, and some to the overlap of related memory traces. Schacter (2001) discusses the major types of error that can cause distortions in memory. Offer, Kaiz, Howard, and Bennett (2000) report a number of significant differences between original responses and subsequent recall when they reinterviewed a group of 48-year-old men about items they were original asked about when they were 12 years old. While *false memories* involve errors in recall, déjà vu experiences involve errors in recognition.

13. Alcoholic blackouts provide a good illustration of the difference between working and permanent memory, as individuals with this condition are fully aware of what they are doing while they are drinking but cannot subsequently recall what happened.

The level of alcohol in their brain tissues presumably blocks the transfer of information from short-term to long-term memory.

14. Restak (1995) notes that adults lose about 10 percent of their neurons during their lifetime, which probably explains some of the cognitive changes associated with normal aging. Unlike most of the other cells of the body, the majority of neurons do not regenerate or get replaced when they die. This may have to do with the fact that their function lies primarily in the connectivity they have developed with other neurons, not in their intrinsic cellular activity. Their unique pattern of synaptic connections cannot necessarily be replicated by a newly formed replacement that does not have the same experiential history.

15. Schacter (1996) reviews the mechanisms involved in strategic and associative retrieval.

16. Damasio (1994) discusses the role of the prefrontal cortex in organizing our mental life. The topic is discussed further in Chapter 15.

17. Cohen (1996) argues that human memory should be studied more often in natural settings, since laboratory experiments limit what can be studied. Her observations on prospective memory are derived from a naturalistic study.

CHAPTER 6. THE IMPACT OF CONSCIOUSNESS

1. The last few years have witnessed an increasing interest in consciousness by a variety of disciplines, including cognitive psychology, philosophy, neuroscience, and artificial intelligence. It is a topic that many people had previously thought was beyond the reach of human understanding, since an entity could not study itself. Recent discussion can be found in: Baars (1997), Chalmers (1996), Churchland (1996), Crick (1994), Damasio (1999), Dennett (1991), Edelman (1992), Greenfield (1995), Greenfield (2000), Humphrey (1992), Mandler (1997), McGinn (1999), Ornstein (1991), and Penrose (1994).

2. Wilkes (1988) argues that terms like *consciousness* are arbitrary and ambiguous as used in common discourse and thus of little use in scientific inquiry. She points out that the word did not exist in English prior to the seventeenth century and was not included in ancient Greek or Chinese writings. She observes that many other languages still lack an equivalent term or anything that corresponds roughly to it. Damasio (1999) points out that *consciousness* and *conscience* initially had overlapping meanings. Although they are now separate words in English and German, they are still combined in Romance languages, such as French and Portuguese. He notes that the first recorded use of the English word *consciousness* was in 1632 and that we still retain the word *unconscionable* to refer to behavior that violates moral or ethical standards.

3. The evolutionary origins of consciousness are discussed in Chapter 8.

4. The question of animal consciousness has been reviewed by a various authors. Griffin (1984) states: "Ethologists and comparative psychologists have discovered increasing complexities in animal behavior during the past few decades. The flexibly and appropriateness of such behavior suggests not only that complex processes occur

within animal brains, but that these events may have much in common with our own mental experiences." Masson and McCarthy (1995) believe that "there are few feelings that apes do not share with us, except perhaps self-hatred. They experience and express exuberance, joy, guilt, remorse, disdain, disbelief, awe, sadness, wonder, tenderness, loyalty, anger, distrust, and love." Radner and Radner (1989) believe that although animals certainly experience pleasurable and painful situations, their subjective experience is not the same as human consciousness. The authors point out that, until fairly recent times, animals were regarded as behaving without any evidence of intention or rational consideration and that theologians thought that it was God's will that man have domination over them. Ristau (1991) reasons that animals think and have conscious awareness because of the complexity of their behavior, their ability to communicate, and their ability to feign injury. She describes a trained African Grey parrot that is able to identify, request, refuse, categorize, and quantify more than 80 different objects. Rogers (1997) thinks that animals have some forms of consciousness and that we should give them the benefit of the doubt about its extent as long as this is not disproven. Although she believes that all vertebrates feel pain, at least as judged by their reactions to being hurt, she questions whether they feel love, hatred, happiness, and sadness in the same way we do. Dennett (1996) offers a more philosophical discussion about the differences between the minds of human and those of other species.

5. The television analogy is from Buckminster Fuller (1973).

6. Bennett (1997) explores the relationship between conscious mental activities and known brain functions.

7. Putting our thoughts into words enables us to see the gaps and contradictions in our understanding of a subject, which is one of the reasons teaching is such a good way of learning. Requiring patients to put their thoughts into order so as to tell their story is one of the ways therapy helps people understand themselves better.

8. Maslow (1970) postulated a hierarchy of needs that prioritize human activities: (1) biological needs, such as hunger, thirst, and sex; (2) safety needs; (3) affiliative needs, such as love and belonging; (4) esteem needs; and (5) self-actualization needs, such as self-fulfillment and achieving one's potential. In many ways, the same sort of priorities help determine the content of consciousness.

9. Children are not held to be legally responsible for their actions because they are considered to be too bound to the immediate present to be able to freely choose what they do. Severely disturbed or demented individuals may also be adjudicated not guilty by reason of insanity if they are unable to appreciate the wrongful *consequences* of their actions.

10. Armstrong (1996) reviews the stories contained in the Book of Genesis.

11. Anna Freud (1946) provides the classic account of psychological defense mechanisms.

12. In Zen, the intent is to stop conceptualizing while fully awake, so that ordinary thoughts are placed in abeyance for a while. Suspending attachment to worldly desires, hopes, and wants is a critical part of the experience. Crook (1980) refers to Zen as a here-and-now, non-duality affair. Orme (1969) points out that "yoga functions by ob-

taining a freedom from memory, that is time, which is accomplished through rhythmic respirations that are supposed to harmonize in some way with the rhythm of the *Great Time.*"

13. Eckblad (1981) distinguishes between behavior that is motivated to achieve some extrinsic goal and behavior that is intrinsically motivated, that is, enjoyable in itself. He believes that there are two distinct cognitive states, one is which a person is motivated by external factors and the other in which one is completely absorbed in what one is doing, during which "the person becomes one with the task and is not aware of anything else. Behavior is not performed as a means to some other end, and is disrupted whenever the person starts to think about ulterior motives or goals for the activity." He compares these states to Maslow's "peak experience" and to Csikszentmihalyi's "flow," in both of which the same complete absorption in the activity is present, as well as a loss of the sense of time and of the feelings of self-awareness and goal-orientation.

CHAPTER 7. EMOTION AS INFORMATION

1. There is little agreement about what emotions are and what they do. Frijda (1986) and Solomon (1976) view them from a psychological perspective; McNaughton (1989) and LeDoux (1996) from a biological one; Ortony, Clore and Collins (1988) and Martin and Clore (2001) from a cognitive one; Plutchik (1980 & 2001) from an evolutionary one; and De Sousa (1987), Lyons (1980), and Sartre (1971) from a philosophical one. General overviews can be found in Eckman and Davidson (1994), Evans (2001), Lazarus and Lazarus (1994), and Lewis and Haviland-Jones (2000). Mayne and Bonanno (2001) review current emotional research.

2. Johnston (1999) refers to the sense of pleasantness or unpleasantness that accompanies a feeling state as its *hedonic tone*, which he uses to denote its evaluative aspect rather than the quality of the experienced sensation. He notes that emotions and somatic sensations share the same range of hedonic tones and that both have been molded by their adaptive value during the course of evolution. McGuire and Troisi (1998) believe that "emotions turn out to be critical information sources that contribute to behavior modulation and strategy modification, primarily in the service of achieving goals."

3. A number of authors propose that emotions provide information about our relationship with the environment. Ortony, Clore, and Collins (1988) note that "the primary function of emotion is to provide information about some special harm or benefit that inheres in the relationship between the person and the environment." Damasio (1994) claims that "feelings are the sensors for the match or lack thereof between our nature (inherited and acquired) and our circumstances." Frijda (1988) states that "emotions arise in response to events that are important to the individual's goals, motives, or concerns." Sartre (1971) contends that "emotions represent a specific manner of apprehending the world." Nussbaum (2001) believes that emotions are judgments of value that appraise whether external objects are salient for our own well-being. Oatley (1992) refers to emotions as "*control signals* that are simpler, cruder and

evolutionarily older than semantic messages." He sees them as part of a monitoring mechanism that evaluates events and responds to change by signaling the cognitive system to respond. Scherer, Schorr, and Johnstone (2001) review the various appraisal theories of emotion.

4. Bentham (1789) lists the following sources of positive feelings: "senses, wealth, skill, friendship, good reputation, power, piety, benevolence, malevolence, memory, imagination, expectation, association, and relief of pain," and the following sources of unpleasant ones: "privation, awkwardness, enmity, ill name, piety, and malevolence."

5. Ryff and Singer (2001) observe that a considerable amount of our life revolves around our relationships with other people, which is why so many of our emotions belong in the affiliative category—and why they arouse our greatest joys and sorrows. Brothers (1997) believes that emotions evolved as social constructs designed to convey nonverbal information between individuals.

6. Some of the emotions that do not fit into the present categories are acceptance, admiration, adoration, amazement, amusement, anguish, appreciation, approval, bewilderment, boredom, chagrin, condemnation, courage, curiosity, determination, discomfort, disdain, disappointment, dissatisfaction, exasperation, gloating, gratitude, greed, horror, indignation, interest, loneliness, outrage, relief, reproach, resignation, smugness, sullenness, surprise, and thankfulness.

7. Ben-Ze'ev (2000) notes that it is the personal meaning and significance that determines the magnitude of the emotional response, rather than the objective magnitude of the stimulus that arouses it.

8. Dehaene (1997) points out that John Von Neuman, one of the founding fathers of computer science, believed that the brain was a mixed analog-digital machine in which analog and digital codes were seamlessly integrated. Clocks and watches with dials are analog devices that gauge the passage of time by the position of their hands in relation to an agreed-upon standard, as also are old-fashioned balance scales which weight objects by comparing them to a series of standard weights. The role of internal reference standards in the production of emotional states is only inferred, however, based on the fact that the type of information conveyed by emotional states resembles the output produced by such comparisons. Hume (1739) observes: "all kinds of reasoning consist in nothing but a *comparison*, and a discovery of those relations, either constant or inconstant, which two or more objects bear each other."

9. Incoming sensory information is relayed from the thalamus to the limbic system, which activates the hypothalamus and the autonomic nervous system in ways that enable "emergency" emotions like fear and anger to generate almost instantaneous responses. Incoming sensory information is also relayed to the sensory cortex and then transmitted to the association and prefrontal areas for appraisal. These areas can then generate emotional responses through their connections back to the limbic system. Patients with prefrontal damage can experience basic emotions, such as fear and anger, but are unable to generate emotions that require cognitive appraisal. Those with significant limbic system damage, on the other hand, are not able to generate either type of

emotional reaction. LeDoux (1996) reviews research concerning the central role of amygdala in generating fear responses.

10. Goleman (1995) popularized the concept of emotional intelligence and stressed its importance in our everyday lives. The concept was first developed in the early 1990s as a specialized component of general intelligence that contributes to an individual's overall success and adaptation.

11. Landman (1993) outlines the role that regret plays in learning from past mistakes and points out how *anticipated regret* can be useful in decision making. She contrasts Harry Truman's view: "Never waste a minute on regret; it's a waste of time," with Santayana's famous dictum: "Those who cannot remember the past are condemned to repeat it."

12. Love is a complex emotional state that involves a cognitive appraisal that matches our perception of a particular individual to some kind of internalized ideal, and thereby generates positive expectations about the future outcome of the relationship. Even when lifelong, the attachment other animals have for each other seems to be much more biologically determined.

13. It is possible that some deeply ingrained moral values, such as the incest taboo, have been determined through natural selection.

14. Solomon (2000) contrasts reason and emotion, where reason is seen as a rational and orderly human achievement and emotion as a capacity for irrational and impulsive behavior that needs to be tamed in order to have civilized societies. De Sousa (1987) reviews the relationship between emotion and rationality, and Langer (1998) discusses the importance of art and esthetics in human affairs.

15. Picard (1997) reviews the issues involved in making computers that can recognize, process, experience, and communicate emotional information. She believes that computers will need the ability to recognize and express emotions in order to be genuinely intelligent and interact naturally with humans.

16. Freud (1930) observes: "Men are beginning to perceive that all this newly won power over space and time, this conquest of the forces of nature, has not increased the amount of pleasure they can obtain in life, has not made them any happier."

17. Kramer (1988) defines music as "discernible patterns of sound over time that are generally experienced as pleasurable by people in a particular culture or subculture." Storr (1992) points out that the origins of music are unclear. Rhythmic singing, chanting, and dancing almost certainly preceded the development of musical instruments, as all known people have such communal practices. Boorstin (1992) observes that music has always been closely associated with religious rituals, mostly as an accompaniment of recitations and other vocal ceremonies. Songs were ways of organizing and remembering stories that were passed down from generation to generation. Until the eighteenth century, musical performances were almost entirely used to accompany singing, either as preludes to or in arrangements for vocal music. Modern instrumental concerts date from that era, thanks to the likes of Bach, Mozart, and Beethoven. Thomas (1995) notes that the origin of music was a favorite topic of

eighteenth-century French writers, most of whom believed that both music and language had their origins in the vocalizations that our ancestors used to communicate feeling states to each other. Hoffman (1997) describes the origins of various musical forms and instruments.

18. Wallin, Merker, and Brown (2000) believe that *measured* music (i.e., music with an isochronous temporal pulse) is universal, often being associated with collective activities such as dancing, and they point out that in Africa there is no word for nonmeasured music (i.e., music you cannot dance to). They note that repetition, a frequently used device in music, produces a high sense of expectancy of what is going to come next. The time sequence of notes (i.e., melody) plays only a small part in Middle Eastern and Asian music, which can make it seem boring to a Western ear. Emotions are chiefly conveyed in music by the tempo, pitch, and intensity of the sounds that are produced, elements similar to the ones used to express emotional tone in spoken language and nonverbal vocalizations. Barrow (1998) believes that the same progression from predictability to surprise takes place in painting and other visual arts.

CHAPTER 8. THE EVOLUTION OF HUMAN BEHAVIOR

1. General portrayals of human evolution can be found in Diamond (1992), Dobzhansky (1962), Eiseley (1946), Goldsmith (1991), Leakey (1994), and Tattersall (1998). Evolutionary theory has become a central tenet of biological science because of its ability to explain why plants and animals are the way they are. Darwin's insights into how we evolved have, however, only recently begun to be incorporated into the sciences of human behavior, where they form an intellectual bridge between psychology and biology, as exemplified by Wilson's (1975) account of sociobiology and Wright's (1995) outline of evolutionary psychology.

2. Dawkins (1976) conceives of biological evolution as a process in which animals are machines that are created by their genes in order for the genes to promote their own survival. He believes that, although genes are inherently selfish in this, there are circumstances when they can best achieve their goals by fostering a limited form of altruism.

3. Pinker (1997) observes that "our brains are adapted to a long-vanished way of life, not to brand-new agricultural and industrial civilizations. They are not wired to cope with anonymous crowding, schooling, written language, government, police courts, armies, modern medicine, formal social institutions, high technology, and other newcomers to the human experience." Burke and Ornstein (1995) provide an overview of the adverse consequences of human technological achievements from antiquity through the present.

4. Kuper (1994) discusses how the transition that gave rise to modern humans was marked by a range of cultural changes that sharply differentiated modern humans from their predecessors. These changes included the ability to fabricate a wide array of fine tools, build shelters, decorate objects, create cave paintings, make jewelry, and carve shapes of animals and humans, all of which indicate the development of a significant capacity for processing symbolic information. Bickerton (1990) believes that these were

the first people to possess recognizable human language. Service (1962 & 1975) points out that so-called primitive cultures are cultures that long ago adapted to a particular environment and have continued into modern times as a result of isolation. Shostak (1983) provides an account of the !Kung San people as told through the day-to-day life of one of its female members.

5. There are few pure cultures left in which everyone shares exactly the same beliefs, since most cultural legacies are now received from a variety of sources. Dawkins (1976) introduced the concept of the "meme," as a unit of cultural replication comparable to the gene, everyone's particular cultural inheritance being determined by the particular combination of memes they receive. Blackmore (1999) elaborates on this concept and indicates how memes and genes (i.e., nature and nurture) interact and combine to form the phenotype on which natural selection operates, with both surviving and replicating when the phenotypic response is adaptive. Feinman and Manzanilla (2000) and Geertz (1973) provide more general information about culture and cultural evolution.

6. Frazer (1950) and Murray (1968) explore the nature and origins of mythology. Myths and folklore passed down from generation to generation were part of the way early mankind interpreted and understood the world. These stories and rituals were always plausible, since they were built on explanations that could not easily be disproved by the events people experienced.

7. Freud (1913) describes animism as follows: "The highly remarkable view of nature and the universe adopted by the primitive races that peoples the world with innumerable spiritual beings, both benevolent and malignant; and these spirits and demons they regard as the causes of natural phenomena, and they believe that not only animals and plants but all the inanimate objects of the world are animated by them."

8. De Lys (1957) describes over three hundred superstitions that various groups still believe to be true.

9. Jaynes (1976) outlines the evidence that supports his thesis. Early forms of consciousness probably began to develop about the same time as early syntactical language, with both likely emerging from more rudimentary prototypes about 40,000 years ago.

10. Wrangham and Peterson (1996) point out that recent studies have shown that bands of chimpanzees at times fight and kill members of other chimpanzee bands, apparently over territory; however, dominance and submission fights within a social group are generally not deadly; only fights between social groups. Instances of lethal aggression among the members of a species have also been reported for gorillas, lions, and spotted hyenas, with several aggressors ganging up to bite and hit the victim—since they have no other weapons.

11. Diamond (1997), Ghiglieari (1999), and Wrangham and Peterson (1996) elaborate on the role of violence in human evolution.

12. Armstrong (1993) provides a scholarly review of the origins of Judaism and Islam.

13. Wilson (1998) observes that "people must belong to a tribe; they yearn to have

a purpose larger than themselves. We are obliged by the deepest drives of the human spirit to make ourselves more than animated dust, and we must have a story to tell about where we came from, and why we are here."

CHAPTER 9. THE GIFT OF LANGUAGE

1. The study of language has become a focus of increased interdisciplinary attention involving psychology, computer science, linguistics, philosophy, and neuroscience. Bickerton (1990 & 1995), Deacon (1997), and Pinker (1994 & 1999) outline these developments for the general reader.

2. Language is a *system* of representational symbols. A symbol is an arbitrary, noniconic signal that uniquely represents some other entity. The flag is a symbol, since it represents (symbolizes) our thoughts and feelings about our nation, but a photograph is just an icon, and nonverbal gestures are just signals. Although some other animals appear to be able to decode certain individual symbols, they do not have the capacity to string them together into a system.

3. Diamond (1997) maintains that there are over five thousand known languages, almost one-fifth of which are spoken in New Guinea where the high mountains have kept populations isolated from each other for centuries. About half of the currently existing languages are threatened with extinction because of the dwindling numbers of people who still speak them.

4. Wolfgang (1979) reviews nonverbal communication. Although there is generally a congruence between the verbal and nonverbal information individuals convey to each other, there can be a discrepancy between the two. This was the basis for the now-discredited *double-bind* theory of schizophrenia, in which the mother was supposed to say one thing to the child verbally while expressing an opposite message emotionally.

5. Darwin (1872) maintains that the precursors of human language can be found in other animals. Noble and Davidson (1996) and Tomasello (1999) discuss the language abilities of other species.

6. The meaning of *man bites dog* is different from *dog bites man* because of the order of the words. Chomsky (1980) notes: "Universal grammar refers to genetically determined properties that are characteristic components of the human biological endowment." This innate ability "enables the child to interpret certain events as linguistic experience and to construct a system of rules and principles on the basis of this experience." Pinker (1994) also believes that we have an in-built predisposition to learn to speak: "Language is a complex, specialized skill which develops in the child spontaneously, without conscious effort or formal instruction, is developed without awareness of its underlying logic, is qualitatively the same in every individual, and is distinct from more general abilities to process information and behave intelligently."

7. Tomasello (1999) observes that children between the ages of one and three are normally "imitation machines" that learn the meaning of words not just by mimicking others but by understanding the accompanying behavioral and attention strategies of the person who is talking. Autistic children appear to lack this ability to understand other persons as intentional agents. Weiskrantz (1988) also provides information about

language development. Silver and Hagan (1990) offer an overview of the learning disabilities that can impair language skills in otherwise normal children.

8. Dehaene (1997) reviews how the brain handles numbers. Mathematics, like writing, requires written symbols to be able to develop its various constructs. Weber (1999) points out that Arabic numerals were introduced into the West by Leonardo Fibonacci, a Pisan mathematician, in 1202. It was hard to compute with the roman numerals that preceded them, as they do not provide any way to multiply or divide and do not have a zero.

9. Deacon (1997) believes that the expansion of the forebrain that made symbolic language possible probably did not reach completion until the time when anatomically modern Homo sapiens began to demonstrate other types of symbol-dependent behaviors, 40,000–45,000 years ago. Lieberman (1991) observes that the position of the larynx in Neanderthal skeletons is like that of current apes, making it likely that they did not develop more than a rudimentary system of vocal communication, which may explain why they disappeared about 35,000 years ago.

10. Bickerton (1990) maintains that language is primarily a representational system and only secondarily for communication. The language structure and grammar of nonindustrialized people are far more complex than the formative talk of young children, even though relatively limited in vocabulary. Pinker (1994) points out that all of our current languages probably have a common origin that dates back to a time before the Aborigines moved to Australia, 40,000–50,000 years ago. How our current languages branched off in different directions after that can be partly traced by examining the ways in which their words and rules are related.

11. The origins of writing date back to the cuneiform script that the Sumerians used to write on clay tablets about 6,000 years ago. Diamond (1997) believes that the first letters were probably stylized representations of familiar objects whose names began with the respective sound. The word *alphabet*, for instance, is derived from the first two letters of the Semitic languages, *aleph* meaning ox and *bet* meaning house, which were at first likely stylized representations of these entities.

CHAPTER 10. THE DEVELOPMENT OF SYMBOLIC THOUGHT

1. Gopnik, Melzoff, and Kuhl (1999), Greenspan (1997), Kagan (1984), Morgan (1995), and Rutter and Rutter (1993) provide accounts of research in infant and child development for the general reader. Harris (1995) offers a more specialized outline of the clinical conditions that occur when brain development goes awry. Bruer (1999) reviews what is actually known about brain development during the first years of life, noting that much of what is being disseminated to the public overstates current research results in ways that may be harmful.

2. Bruer (1999) points out that a child's brain reaches almost adult size by age six or seven, by which time it is more than three times larger than it was at birth, whereas an ape's brain grows only about 30–40 percent after birth. The relative immaturity of the human infant's brain is the main reason we are so helpless at birth and are so sensitive to environmental influences during the first few years of life.

3. Genetic evolution is parsimonious and usually involves just enough change in DNA to achieve the desired adaptation under the species' usual living circumstances. Geese, for instance, are genetically encoded to follow the first moving object they see—as this will ordinarily be their mother—rather than being encoded to follow the mother *per se*, which presumably would require a more complicated genetic message. As a result, they can become imprinted on humans and follow them, rather than their mother, if the human happens to be the first moving object they come across (Lorentz, 1981).

4. Various stages of child development are described by Cullingford (1999), Dunn (1988), Kagan (1978), and McShane (1991). Piaget and Inhelder (1969) formulate four stages of cognitive development: (1) *sensorimotor*, from birth until about two, during which the child lacks true thoughts, lives in the present, and connects motor responses to sensory input, (2) *pre-operational*, from two until six or seven, marked by the transition to representing reality mentally, (3) *concrete operations*, from six or seven until twelve or thirteen, when the child can understand the principle of conservation, and (4) *formal operations*, from thirteen on, which marks the ability to reason about concrete visible events, think hypothetically, and entertain ideas of what is possible about the world. Vygotsky (1978) notes that the creation of an imaginary situation is not a fortuitous act in a child's life but rather a means of developing abstract thought. He believes that "once children learn how to use the planning function of their language effectively, a view of the future becomes an integral part of their approaches to their surroundings."

5. Hass (1970) notes that curiosity is a characteristic of nonspecialized creatures that are able to adapt to various circumstances rather than being fitted for a very specific way of life. Grown-up individuals unfortunately tend to lose a great deal of their curiosity about the world.

6. Imitative learning is generally not recallable, because it occurs outside of conscious awareness. It can thus shape our behavior without our knowing it.

7. According to de Waal (1996), chimpanzees, orangutans, and young children can recognize a spot that has been painted on their forehead as being on themselves when they see it in a mirror, since they try to wipe it off—indicating they have developed some type of mental self-representation. Monkeys, however, are unable to do this.

8. Young children initially make mistakes in forming categories, like using the word *moon* to represent oranges, lamps, balloons, and crescent-shaped objects. The *Similarities* subtest of the Wechsler Intelligence Scale for Children, Third Edition (WISC-III) asks the subject whether different objects belong to the same or different categories, for instance, "In what way are an apple and an orange alike?" Children with limited symbolic processing abilities do not perform well on this test.

9. Morality involves a conscious appraisal of a given act and a sense that one is free to choose between alternatives. De Waal (1996) argues that some aspects of morality are recognizable in other animals, including instances of apparent empathy, giving, revenge, and peacemaking. Kagan (1998), while acknowledging that chimpanzees may possess rules and punish fellow chimpanzees who break them, does not believe he will

ever see a guilty chimpanzee, since guilt requires "the ability to infer the state of others, reflect on past actions, compare the products of that reflection with acquired standards, realize that a particular action that violated a standard could have been inhibited, and evaluate the self as a consequence of that violation."

10. Kagan (1984) believes that infants create composite schemas of what they have experienced and then focus attention on discrepancies between these internal representations and what they perceive. He calls this the *discrepancy principle* and explains that "the mind grows at the edge where the expected does not occur or is moderately transformed."

11. Johnson, Cohen, Brown, Smailes, and Bernstein (1999) found that abused and neglected children were more than four times as likely as other children to develop personality disorders in early adult life.

12. Greenspan (1997) believes that we are in danger of losing our cohesion as a society because of our lack of attention to emotional development in infants and young children. He is concerned that, as more and more young children spend significant amounts of time in group day care, they will have far less opportunity for one-to-one relationships with adults. He believes that unless a child masters the level of two-way intentional communication normally achieved by an eight-month-old infant, its language, cognitive, psychosexual, and social patterns will ultimately develop in a piecemeal and disorganized manner.

13. Bowlby (1973) stresses the importance of attachment in human development. Gopnik, Melzoff, and Kuhl (1999) note that bonding between infant and caregiver is essential for normal human development, as "no creature spends more time dependent on others for its very existence than a human baby, and no creature takes on the burden of that dependence so long and so readily as a human adult." Kagan (1984) observes that children are apparently born with distinctive temperamental traits which are subsequently reinforced or modified by how well they fit with their caregiver's expectations and tolerance. Temperamental qualities, such as caution/timidity and sociability/fearlessness, tend to persist from the first birthday to late childhood, so that the very shy, very timid six-year-old is likely to become an adolescent who is quiet and tense with strangers.

14. Dunn (1988) observes that children start managing their social world during their second and third year, during which time they learn how to get attention and cooperation, cope with disagreements, understand another individual's intentions, and provide comfort for someone in distress. During the ensuing years, they gradually develop the ability to interpret and anticipate other people's reactions, understand the relationships between other individuals, and comprehend the sanctions and accepted practices of their world.

15. Candland (1993) reviews what is known about feral children discovered during the eighteenth and nineteenth centuries. These unsocialized children were of great interest back then because it was thought that they could reveal which aspects of human behavior were innate and which learned. Studying them did not settle these questions, however, since no one could be sure whether they had been raised by animals

or simply abandoned by their parents because they were retarded. Spitz's (1946) studies of young infants raised in institutions show how important psychological attachment is for a child's well-being.

CHAPTER 11. THE CONCEPT OF TIME

1. Davies (1996), Friedman (1990), Morris (1985), Toulmin and Goodfield (1965), and Whitrow (1972 & 1989) provide general accounts of how the concept of time has changed. More specialized books about time include philosophical approaches by Baert (2000), Butterfield (1999), Fraser, Haber, and Muller (1972), Holland (1999), Orme (1969), Poidevin and MacBeath (1993), and Shallis (1983), and psychological ones by Block (1990), Bradshaw and Szabadi (1997), Brown (1996), Flaherty (1999), Gorman and Wessman (1972), Helfrich (1996), Ornstein (1997), Rappaport (1990), and Slife (1993).

2. Newton (1642–1727) refers in his *Principia* to "absolute, true and mathematical time, which of itself, and from its own nature, flows equably without relation to anything external." Leibniz (1646–1716), his contemporary, did not agree that moments of time can exist independently of events and argued that we derive time from our experience that events which are not simultaneous occur in a particular order, one after the other. Although Newton's ideas prevailed for almost three centuries, Leibniz's position proved to be closer to the modern view (Whitrow, 1989).

3. Nichols (1891) observes: "Time has been called an act of mind, of reason, of perception, of intuition, of sense, of memory, of will, and of all possible compounds and compositions to be made of these." James (1890) notes that "awareness of *change* is the condition on which our perception of time's flow depends, but the *experience* of time cannot simply be explained on the basis of our perception of such changes."

4. Zaleski (1994) notes that the French philosopher Guyau wrote in 1890 that time is "a strategy of coping with the world; our consciousness of time is a side effect of goal-oriented behavior; time is a product of consciousness. Whereas the present is perceived, the past and future are represented."

5. Bates, Elman, and Li (1994) describe the developing child's changing concept of time. Piaget (1927) points out that even though young children may know how old they are, they do not have a conception of time until they are seven or eight. This is apparent when a five year-old is asked how old a sibling or friend is, and then questioned about which one of them was born first or what their age difference will be when they are grown up. Hall (1983) reports that the Hopi and Sioux Indians do not have a word for time, that verbs in the Hopi language do not have any tenses, and that concepts of past, present and future simply do not exist for them. According to him, the Navajo also live in an eternal present where the future is so unreal to them that they are neither interested in nor motivated by future rewards. Lee (1950) reports that the Trobriand Islanders also have no tenses, no linguistic distinction between past and present, no causal relationships, and no equivalent of *why* or *because* in their language. Events and objects are self-contained, they do not *become* something else—so that a fruit does not become ripe, it just passes into a different entity, a *ripe fruit*. Gell (1992), however, does

not believe people in different cultures experience time in markedly different ways, even though their way of describing it may differ.

6. Seddon (1987) claims that "time is just a matter of relationship between events. Human experience is composed of a ceaselessly changing panorama of events, some of which occur earlier and some later than others. We can arrange them in a temporal sequence, but we cannot state which occur in the past, the present or the future except in relation to an arbitrarily chosen point of reference."

7. Viorst describes how we grow and change, for better or worse, as we deal with the inevitable losses that we encounter as we progress from childhood through old age. Novey (1968) argues that: "The very concept of history as a predictive instrument suggests that today's views of history will influence tomorrow's course of events. The existence of optimistic or pessimistic outlooks is significantly based on the appraisal of past events, and such mood states bear considerably on what will actually happen tomorrow."

8. The moon actually takes 29.5306 days to complete its rotation around the earth and the earth 365.2422 days to complete its cycle around the sun, which averages about 12.37 lunar months per year. A day is the period of rotation of the earth around its own axis, that rotation being what makes it seem that the sun rotates across the sky. We arbitrarily divide the day into 24 hours, each containing 60 minutes, each 60 seconds long, and then calibrate our clocks to measure them. Because the earth moves with varying speeds in its orbit at different times of the year, and because the plane of the earth's equator is at an incline to its orbital plane, the actual length of the solar day differs at different times of the year. To standardize our time so that it is not subject to these variations, one second is now defined as 9,192,631,770 beats of a cesium atom, rather than 1/86,400 of a day. What we measure either way is, of course, only *earth* time. If intelligent creatures exist elsewhere in the universe, their sense of time will be unique to their location (Aveni, 1989). The various inventions our ancestors developed to record and measure the passage of time are described by Aveni (1989), Borst (1993), Richards (1998), and Whitrow (1989).

9. Whitrow (1972) observes that the development of mechanical clocks in medieval Europe did not spring from a desire to register the passage of time but rather from a monastic demand for accurate determination of the hours when the various religious offices and prayers should be said. The first clocks had no dials and merely sounded a bell on the hour, a tradition many churches continue to this day. Early church clocks, although often elaborate, were not particularly accurate, and were not synchronized from one town to the next. Two mid-seventeenth-century inventions—the pendulum clock and the minute hand—made timing mechanisms more exact and reliable. In 1759 John Harrison won the prize that the British government offered for the construction of a chronometer that was accurate enough to determine longitude at sea. This piece of technology opened the oceans for trade and maritime conquest. Richards (1998) details how the Industrial Revolution from 1760 to 1830 led to the increasing urbanization of Western societies as workers moved from the countryside to the cities in search of employment. Urban life became increasingly time scheduled, as industrial jobs were

not coordinated to the rhythm of the seasons that typified farm work. Fewer than 10 percent of Americans had a clock of any kind in their homes in 1790, but this changed dramatically as trains and factories began to proliferate and modern industrial society took center stage.

10. Shapin (1996) quotes the observation of Robert Boyle (1627–1691) about the famous Strasbourg clock, which had been completed in 1574: "The several pieces making up that curious engine are so framed and adapted, and are put into such a motion, that though the numerous wheels, and other parts of it, move several ways, and that without any thing either of knowledge or design; yet each part performs its part in order to the various ends, for which it was contrived, as regularly and uniformly as if it knew and were concerned to do its duty."

11. Whitrow (1972) observes that "the cyclic view of time was associated with the belief that the world was involved in an endless cycle of death and renewal. The cyclic motions of the sun, moon, planets, and stars were thought to determine the outcome of earthly events—and thus became the object of worship. It was generally believed that a correct knowledge of the relative position of the heavenly bodies was necessary for the success of most earthly activities. Brandon (1972) notes that astrology originated about 400 BC in the belief that these *writings of the heavens* indicated a person's destiny.

12. Weber (1999) recounts how dreadful apprehensions of the approaching end were an integral part of the medieval world. Visions of the Apocalypse infused the times with beliefs of the imminence of the Second Coming of Christ in which evil-doers would be destroyed and God would install the kingdom of heaven on earth. Natural disasters, like earthquakes, volcanoes, and comets, were taken as signs that the end was near and were viewed with awe and trepidation. People were not sure whether the world would be destroyed or turned into a paradise.

13. Toulmin and Goodfield (1965) note that Georges Buffon was probably the first to publicly oppose church dogma about the age of the world, with the publication of *Histoire Naturelle* in 1749, in which he claimed that the quantity of marine fossils proved a longer duration. He later retracted his remarks after being censured by the church.

14. Heilbroner (1995) defines *progress* as the idea that "the present is in some fashion superior to the past and, by extension, that the future will be superior to the present." Sebba (1972) observes: "The breakdown of the medieval world-view initiated a radical change in the Western concept and experience of self. Rather than being helpless passengers aboard the earth, people began to see themselves as actors who could effect change on the world around them."

15. As Brandon (1972) points out, "time sense . . . has a kind of debit side—mankind has to pay a price for this faculty that has made him so successful biologically in the struggle for existence. Because of their ability to look forward in time, every man and woman is aware that they are subject to the process of decay and ultimately, death. Although their time-sense enables them to secure themselves against the contingencies that threaten their material well-being and [to] improve the material conditions of their life, it also makes them aware of their ultimate insecurity."

16. Melges (1990) observes that without a sense of time perspective, individuals

are not able to experience their own identity. He reports that experimental subjects given THC (the active ingredient of marijuana) lose both their sense of identity and their sense of time. Rappaport (1990) believes that temporal disturbances underlie most addictive disorders. He reports that addicts tend to have difficulty dealing with "empty," unfilled time when there is "nothing to do," as well as difficulty conceiving of what to do in the future and how to spend their spare time to enhance it.

17. Becker (1996) remarks that "human capital analysis starts with the assumption that individuals decide on their education, training, medical care, and other additions to knowledge and health by weighing the benefits and costs. Benefits include cultural and other nonmonetary gains along with improvement in earnings and occupations, while costs usually depend mainly on the foregone value of the time spent on these investments."

18. Sharp (1981) notes that economics is concerned with the time that human beings have at their disposal and how they allocate it between alternative activities: "If men knew how to go about it, they would try to spend their lifelong ration of time so that it would yield them the maximum amount of happiness."

CHAPTER 12. SCIENCE AND RELIGION AS WAYS OF KNOWING

1. Benz (2000) maintains that science and religion are entirely compatible approaches to experiencing reality, one subjective and the other objective. He maintains that they address different kinds of truth and have different kinds of answers. Feynman (1998) believes, however, that science and religion have an inherent conflict, because "while science teaches us to doubt what we see and are told, religion teaches us to believe with certainty."

2. Medin and Atran (1999) observe: "Religion and magic were such intricate parts of everyday life that these explanatory systems, often with explicit causal mechanisms, were called upon to fill in unknown details of disease transmission and other misfortune. The availability of this powerful explanatory framework could go so far as to override or supplant more implicitly held theories about general biological phenomena. People then, like people today, wanted satisfying and explicit answers to help them understand the often overwhelming dramas of everyday life, and their religion often offered explanations invoking all-powerful agents whose scope of efficacy left few phenomena unexplained."

3. Galileo Galilei (1564–1642) was one of the founders of modern science. A physicist, mathematician, and astronomer, he was forced by the church to recant the heliocentric views outlined in his *Dialogue on the Two Chief World Systems*, and he spent the rest of his life under house arrest.

4. Desroche (1979) notes how the established order wanted to preserve itself by having people renounce worldly hopes of betterment in favor of the promise of religious salvation. He quotes Pope Leo XIII in 1882: "Finally the question of the relations of the rich and the poor, with which economists are so concerned, would be completely resolved in that it would be well established that poverty is not without dignity, that the rich man should be merciful and generous and the poor man should be content with his

lot and his work, and the one must get to heaven through patience and the other through generosity."

5. The trouble that less developed countries experience when they try to change from an authoritarian system to a more democratic one demonstrates how long-held cultural beliefs about matters like individual responsibility, self-determination, and societal organization affect the implementation of beneficial political and economic reforms.

6. Kushner's solution is to believe that God does not get involved in the day-to-day details of our individual lives, just the larger scheme of things. Delbanco (1999) claims that the basic tenet of all religions is to say to the sufferer that their only deliverance is to discover and submit to something larger and more enduring than themselves.

7. The sense that our lives have meaning and purpose seems to depend on being able to find something outside of ourselves which we feel is important enough to invest time and energy in. It can be another person, a good cause, or a transcendent belief, but it gives us a sense of purpose and makes our life seem worth living. Self-preoccupation and pure rationality do not seem able to provide a sense of sustained pleasure or meaning. It seems that to find one's self, one first has to lose oneself in some external object or event.

CHAPTER 13. SHARED EXPECTATIONS

1. Brothers (1997) observes that even our individual sense of *self* is essentially a social construct. Our concept of our own identity is largely determined by the pattern of religious, ethnic, social, occupational, educational, and community groups to which we belong—as well as by the ones to which we do not belong. The need to have an enduring sense of self seems to increase as individuals interact with growing numbers of nonkinship people, for the notion of the individual does not become prominent in Western art and literature until the nineteenth century.

2. Lens and Moreas (1994) point out that, when there is an immediate advantage in each member's acting for personal gain in a way that would be deleterious if all were to do it, individuals can rationalize that one person's behavior will not make much difference, since all the other members will support the group's effort. For instance, it does not make much difference if only one or two people cheat on their income tax returns, drive gas-guzzling vehicles, or discharge toxic wastes into our rivers; but if everyone were to do these things, the whole group would suffer. The Aristotle quotation is from *Politics*, Book II.

3. Rice (1965) maintains that the main functions of leaders are: (a) to articulate a vision of an achievable future that resonates with the aspirations of their followers, (b) to outline a credible way of achieving the goal, and (c) to energize their followers to work towards achieving it. Taking polls to see what the other members want and offering this back to them does not fulfill these functions, as this is really a form of followership. Effective leadership involves inspiring one's followers to sacrifice the fulfillment of some of their individual needs and desires for the sake of the larger whole, a difficult task in today's world, as leaders are no longer trusted in the way they once were.

4. Schumacher (1973) believes that, while the Puritan ethic of communal service balanced personal greed when capitalism first began, individual motivations now run unchecked by such social concerns. The debate about the extent to which markets should be left to run free or be regulated for the common good is far from settled, even as capitalistic practices are currently transforming the global economy.

5. The ability to accumulate goods and possessions was a necessary precursor to the development of barter and trade. Trade did not really begin to flourish until money was invented as a resource that could be easily kept and exchanged. The advent of paper money and modern financial institutions in the seventeenth century greatly enlarged the range of economic endeavors in which people could invest their time and effort—and their hopes.

6. Tiger (1979) describes how the value of a company's shares on the stock market depends on people's *perception* of its future success, noting that economic predictions depend on the amount of confidence investors have about the future of the economy. As Sternsher (1999) points out, "the New Deal years were a time of hope restored, even though economic recovery still had a long way to go." He believes that the New Deal was primarily a political and psychological success.

7. Awbrey (1999) maintains that "there is no consensus, no clear direction for the future. The culture no longer inspires society, and the bonds of shared experience that once held people together are reduced to TV, pro sports, and plotless but visually spectacular movies." Toffler (1970) notes that it is difficult to retain a sense of personal continuity when changes in the culture accelerate too rapidly. The sense of things being out of control tends to lead people to drop out and focus on intensifying the present.

8. Restak (1994) quotes a letter he received from a high school teacher: "In dealing with a high school population of profoundly underachieving adolescent/young adult males between the ages of 14 and 19, we regularly witness students whose attention span, motivation, autonomy and emotion appear diminished if not restricted. Many of these kids lack age appropriate cognitive development as demonstrated by their lack of insight, abstraction, and concept formation, inferential aptitude, organization and planning, and a sense of autonomy."

9. Hughes (1988) discusses the relationship between crime and industrialization in describing how Australia was initially settled.

CHAPTER 14. DESPAIR

1. Despair and depression have been part of the human condition since recorded time. Hippocrates (460–370 BC) recognized their symptoms: "an aversion to food, despondency, sleeplessness, irritability, restlessness, fear and depression which are prolonged." Goodwin and Jamison (1990) offer an overview of depressive and manic-depressive disorders for the professional, while Whybrow (1997) does the same for the general reader. Andrew Solomon (2001) provides a lucid description of the disorder, as well as a personal survey of what is currently known about it.

2. Styron (1990), in writing about his own encounter with depression, comments: "Depression is a disorder of mood, so mysteriously painful and elusive in the way it

becomes known to the self—to the mediating intellect—as to verge close to being beyond description. It thus remains nearly incomprehensible to those who have not experienced it in its extreme mode, although the gloom, 'the blues' which people go through occasionally and associate with the general hassle of everyday existence are of such prevalence that they do give many individuals a hint of the illness in its catastrophic form." Seligman (1991), however, believes that clinical depression is just a more severe form of the ordinary sadnesses and setbacks of everyday life.

3. The symptoms of grief and depression can overlap. Freud (1917) distinguished between what he called *mourning* and *melancholia* by noting that "the fall in self-esteem is absent in grief, but otherwise the features are the same."

4. Whybrow (1997) observes that "seeking ways to blot out variation in mood is equivalent to the ancient mariner throwing away his sextant or the airline pilot ignoring his navigational devices. Emotion is the homeostat of life, an instrument of social self-correction—and when we are happy or sad, it has meaning."

5. Engel (1961) notes that "grief is a characteristic response to the loss of a valued object, be it the loss of a person, a cherished possession, a job, status, home, country, an ideal, a part of the body." Parkes (1972), however, points out that exactly what has been lost is not always clear: "The loss of a husband, for instance, may mean the loss of a sexual partner, companion, accountant, gardener, baby-minder, audience, bed-warmer, and so on. Moreover, it is usually accompanied by a considerable drop in income which means that the widow must sell her house, move to a strange environment and give up her job." Archer (1999) reviews contemporary views of grief.

6. Veninga (1985) offers vignettes that illustrate the varied nature of the grief process.

7. Freud (1917) observes that the task of grief is to detach the memories and expectations of the survivors from the dead. He notes that the work of mourning involves bringing up "each single one of the memories and hopes which bound the libido to the object." Parkes (1972) also notes that grief involves changing one's representations of the loved one.

8. The ancient Greeks thought that depression was caused by an excess of black bile, which is the origin of the word *melan-cholia*. According to Beck (1967), "the central core of depression involves a self that seems worthless, a world that seems meaningless, and a future that seems hopeless." Lewis (1932) discusses how time is experienced differently by patients with depression.

9. O'Keane (2000) summarizes evidence showing that the hypothalamic-pituitary-adrenal axis is activated in depression, as well as in some states that make people vulnerable to it. Brown and Harris (1978) found the following vulnerability factors in a study of depressed English housewives: lack of a job outside the home, absence of a confiding relationship with their husband, three or more children under fourteen, death of their own mother before they were eleven, and low self-esteem.

10. Nesse (1991) reviews various theories about the adaptive function of depressive states. He observes that "clinicians have long noted that depression is common in

people who are pursuing unreachable goals," and points out that "low mood is aroused by a mismatch between achievements and expectations."

11. Kleinman and Good (1985) review cross-cultural studies of depression. Individuals in present-oriented cultures generally experience loss with less grieving and less suffering, possibly because they expect less.

12. Bibring (1953) maintains that individuals become depressed when they believe that they are going to lose their sense of self-esteem. He notes that self-esteem depends on: (a) the need to feel that one is loved, appreciated, or worthy of being noticed; (b) the need to feel strong, superior, or secure; and (c) the need to be good and not hateful or destructive. Supportive treatment should thus, among other things, be directed at helping patients feel that they are appreciated, capable, and worthwhile.

CHAPTER 15. HUMAN NATURE—IT'S ABOUT TIME

1. Wilson (1978) mentions other distinctive behaviors that characterize human societies, including athletic sports, bodily adornment, calendars, cooking, decorative art, etiquette, fire making, funeral rites, incest taboos, laws, marriage, medicines, names, puberty customs, religious rituals, and trade.

2. Horgan believes we gravitate to belief systems whose model of humankind is closest to our own, and our own beliefs about human nature are, in turn, shaped by the groups to which we belong. He maintains that we would not have so many theories of human nature if any one of them could produce factual evidence to support it.

3. It seems that only about 500 of our approximately 35,000 genes are different from those of our closest genetic relative, the chimpanzee. These will be identified once both the human and chimpanzee genomes are fully elucidated, likely within the next decade. Specifying human uniqueness at this molecular level will be a remarkable milestone in the history of mankind. Once it is accomplished, the next step will be to determine exactly what proteins these genes give rise to and what functions they have in the development and operation of the brain, for this is where they will likely have their greatest impact. This will not be a simple task, however, as they will undoubtedly interact with the rest of the genome and with the environment in highly complex ways.

4. Dretske (1988) discusses how intangible entities like reasons, beliefs, desires, purposes, and plans operate in a world of causes to explain human behavior. He attempts to reconcile how thoughts, purposes, intentions, hopes, desires, and fears determine what we do by interfacing with the neurophysiological machinery of the nervous system.

5. One of the major differences between the human and primate prefrontal cortex is the duration of the time intervals they can process. The other primates can integrate only the very recent past and very near future, as measured by the delay tests used to assess prefrontal function. Goldman-Rakic (1984) believes that these tests assess crucial cognitive abilities that depend on the capacity to recognize that an object continues to exist in time and space when it is not in view. Further information about the

prefrontal cortex can be found in: Benson (1994), Fuster (1997), Krasnegor, Lyon, and Goldman-Rakic (1997), and Struss and Benson (1986).

6. Various studies suggest that at least three separate cognitive functions are involved in coordinating future-oriented behaviors: (a) short-term or working memory, (b) anticipatory schemas or sets, and (c) inhibitory control. Working memory and anticipatory sets appear to work together as buffers that can hold relevant retrospective and prospective data *on line* simultaneously to facilitate their use in planning and decision making.

7. Calne (1999) observes that different areas of the prefrontal cortex have primary control of different functions, as is evidenced when they are damaged. Disinhibition and diminished social skills result from damage to the ventromedial prefrontal region, disruption of executive function from damage to the dorsolateral region, and apathy from lesions in the inner aspect of the region between the two lobes.

8. Arnsten (1998) reports that exposure to stress can produce a functional lesion of the prefrontal cortex in monkeys, possibly caused by the high levels of dopamine and norepinephrine that are released in the brain during psychological stress. She also found that these stress-induced impairments could be ameliorated by pretreatment with compounds that block the actions of these neurotransmitters.

9. McKinney (1988) notes that animal models can, however, be useful in understanding certain aspects of human mental illnesses, even if "there is no such thing as a comprehensive animal model for any psychiatric syndrome, identical in terms of etiology, symptoms, underlying mechanisms, and treatment responsiveness." The introduction of a human Alzheimer's disease gene into mice to produce a model of the disorder with comparable brain pathology and memory deficits is an example of the ways that animal models can be made to be useful, both for investigating the causal mechanisms involved in a disorder and for screening effective treatments for it. Andreason (2001) provides an overview of current research in mental illness for the general reader.

10. Barch et al. (2001), for instance, demonstrate selective dorsolateral prefrontal cortex dysfunction in schizophrenia. Individuals with this disorder have difficulty differentiating their internal, reflective information-processing channel from their external, experiential one, so that they mistake imagination for reality, and behave accordingly. Cosgrove (2000) notes that prefrontal lobotomy, in which the connections between the prefrontal cortex and the rest of the brain are surgically severed, was introduced into the United States in the early 1940s as a treatment for this and other severe mental illnesses. While it relieved many of the more acute symptoms, it also resulted in apathy, decreased attention, disinhibition, and significant personality change, much like that produced by other forms of prefrontal damage. According to Cosgrove, more than 50,000 procedures were performed before the use of the procedure waned in response to mounting ethical concerns.

11. Boniecki (1978) believes that mankind needs to focus on more distant horizons, pointing out that currently "man's distant time frame is two years, with the horizon of main interest in his future being correlated to the degree of satisfaction of his immediate (basic) needs."

12. McGinn (1999) questions whether we really would be better off if we had more complete knowledge of ourselves, noting that there is nothing in the concept of knowledge that guarantees it will make us happy. He believes that the bond between the mind and the brain is an ultimate mystery that we will never be able to unravel, since the structure of human intelligence is limited in ways that make it impossible for us ever to understand the way that our thoughts actually determine our actions.

References

Al-Azm, S.J. 1967. *Kant's Theory of Time*. New York: Philosophical Library.

Abramson, L., Metalsky, G., & Alloy, L. 1988. The hopelessness theory of depression: Does the research test the theory. In L. Abramson (Ed.), *Social Cognition and Clinical Psychology*. New York: Guilford Press.

Allman, J.M. 1999. *Evolving Brains*. New York: Scientific American Library.

Anderson S.W., Bechra, A., Damasio, H., Tranel, D., & Damasio, A.R. 1999. Impairment of social and moral behavior related to early damage in human prefrontal cortex. *Nature Neuroscience* 2 (11): 1032–1037.

Andreason, N. 2001. *Brave New Brain: Conquering Mental Illness in the Era of the Genome*. New York: Oxford University Press.

Aquinas, St. T. 1267 (1963). Hope. In *Summa Theologica* Vol. 33. New York: McGraw-Hill.

Archer, J. 1999. *The Nature of Grief: The Evolution and Psychology of Reactions to Loss*. London: Routledge.

Armstrong, K. 1993. *A History of God*. New York: Alfred A. Knopf.

Armstrong, K. 1996. *In the Beginning: The 4000-Year Quest of Judaism, Christianity, and Islam*. New York: Alfred A. Knopf.

Arnsten, A.F.T. 1998. Stress impairs prefrontal cortical function. *Journal of the American Academy of Child and Adolescent Psychiatry* 38 (2): 220–222.

Aveni, A.F. 1989. *Empires of Time: Calendars, Clocks and Cultures*. New York: Bantam Books.

Averill, J.R, Catlin, G., & Chon, K.K. 1990. *Rules of Hope*. New York: Springer-Verlag.

Awbrey, D.S. 1999. *Finding Hope in an Age of Melancholy*. Boston: Little, Brown.

Baars, B.J. 1997. *In the Theater of Consciousness: The Workplace of the Mind*. New York: Oxford University Press.

Baert, P. (Ed.) 2000. *Time in Contemporary Intellectual Thought*. Amsterdam: Elsevier.

Bandura, A. 1997. *Self-Efficacy: The Exercise of Control*. New York: W.H. Freeman.

Barch, D.M., Carter, C.S., Braver, T.S., Sabb, F.W., MacDonald, A., Noll, D.C. & Cohen,

J.D. 2001. Selective deficits in the prefrontal cortex function in medication-naive patients with schizophrenia. *Archives of General Psychiatry* 58:280–288.

Barrow, J.D. 1991. *Theories of Everything: The Quest for Ultimate Explanation.* Oxford: Clarendon Press.

Barrow, J.D. 1998. *Impossibility: The Limits of Science and the Science of Limits.* Oxford: Oxford University Press.

Bates, E., Elman J., & Li, P. 1994. Language in, on, and about time. In Haith, M.M., Benson, J.B., Roberts, R.J., Jr., & Pennington, B.F. (Eds.), *The Development of Future-Oriented Processes.* Chicago: University of Chicago Press.

Bechra, A., Damasio, A., Damasio, H., & Anderson, S. 1994. Insensitivity to future consequences following damage to human prefrontal cortex. *Cognition* 50:7–15.

Beck, A.T. 1967. *The Diagnosis and Management of Depression.* Philadelphia: University of Pennsylvania Press.

Becker, G.S. 1996. *Accounting for Tastes.* Cambridge: Harvard University Press.

Beecher, H.K. 1995. The powerful placebo. *Journal of the American Medical Association* 159: 1602–1606.

Bennett, M.R. 1997. *The Idea of Consciousness: Synapses of the Mind.* Amsterdam: Harwood.

Benson, D.F. 1994. *The Neurology of Thinking.* New York: Oxford University Press.

Bentham, J. 1789 (1970). *An Introduction to the Principles of Morals and Legislation.* J.H. Burns & H.L.A. Hart (Eds). London: Athlone Press.

Benz, A. 2000. *The Future of the Universe: Chance, Chaos, God?* New York: Continuum.

Ben-Ze'ev, A. 2000. *The Subtlety of Emotions.* Cambridge: MIT Press.

Bibring, E. 1953. The mechanism of depression. In P. Greenacre (Ed.), *Affective Disorders.* New York: International Press.

Bickerton, D. 1990. *Language and Species.* Chicago: University of Chicago Press.

Bickerton, D. 1995. *Language and Human Behavior.* Seattle: University of Washington Press.

Bjorklund, D.F. & Pellegrini, A.D. 2002. *The Origins of Human Nature: Evolutionary Developmental Psychology.* Washington, D.C.: American Psychological Association.

Blackmore, S. 1999. *The Meme Machine.* Oxford: Oxford University Press.

Bloch, E. 1986. *The Principle of Hope.* Cambridge: MIT Press.

Block, R.A. (Ed.) 1990. *Cognitive Models of Psychological Time.* Hillsdale: Lawrence Erlbaum.

Boniecki, G. 1978. Is man interested in his future? *International Journal of Psychology* 12:59–64 and 13:219–244.

Boorstin, D.J. 1992. *The Creators.* New York: Random House.

Borst, A. 1993. *The Ordering of Time.* Trans. A. Winnard. Chicago: University of Chicago Press.

Bowlby, J. 1973. *Attachment and Loss.* New York: Basic Books.

Bradshaw, C.M. & Szabadi, E. (Eds.) 1997. *Time and Behavior: Psychological and Neurological Analysis.* Amsterdam: Elsevier.

Brand, S. 1999. *The Clock of the Long Now: Time and Responsibility.* New York: Basic Books.

Brandon, S.G.F. 1972. The deification of time. In J.T. Fraser, F.C. Haber, & G.H. Muller (Eds.), *The Study of Time*. Berlin: Springer-Verlag.

Broadwell, R.D. (Ed.) 1994. *Neuroscience, Memory and Language*. Washington, D.C.: Library of Congress.

Brothers, L. 1997. *Friday's Footprint: How Society Shapes the Human Mind*. New York: Oxford University Press.

Brown, G.W. & Harris, T. 1978. *Social Origins of Depression: A Study of Psychiatric Disorders in Women*. New York: Free Press.

Brown, J. (Ed.) 1976. *Recall and Recognition*. London: John Wiley & Sons.

Brown, J.W. 1996. *Time, Will, and Mental Process*. New York: Plenum.

Bruer, J.T. 1999. *The Myth of the First Three Years: A New Understanding of Early Brain Development and Lifelong Learning*. New York: Free Press.

Bruner, J. 1986. *Actual Minds, Possible Worlds*. Cambridge: Harvard University Press.

Brunner, R.D. 2000. Alternatives to prediction. In D. Sarewitz, R.A. Pielke, Jr., & R. Byerly, Jr. (Eds.), *Prediction: Science, Decision Making and the Future of Nature*. Washington, D.C.: Island Press.

Bruton, H.J. 1997. *On the Search for Well-Being*. Ann Arbor: University of Michigan Press.

Bultmann, R. & Rengstrof, K.H. 1963. *Hope*. London: Adam & Charles Black.

Burke, J. & Ornstein, R. 1995. *The Axemaker's Gift: A Double-Edged History of Human Culture*. New York: G. P. Putnam's Sons.

Burke, P. 2000. *A Social History of Knowledge: From Gutenberg to Diderot*. Malden: Blackwell.

Butterfield, J. (Ed.) 1999. *The Arguments of Time*. Oxford: Oxford University Press.

Byrne, R. 1995. *The Thinking Ape: Evolutionary Origins of Intelligence*. Oxford: Oxford University Press.

Calne, D. 1999. *Within Reason: Rationality and Human Behavior*. New York: Pantheon Books.

Calvin, W. H. 1996. *The Cerebral Code: Thinking Thought in the Mosaics of the Mind*. Cambridge: MIT Press.

Campbell, D. 1997. *The Mozart Effect*. New York: Avon Books.

Candland, D.K. 1993. *Feral Children and Clever Animals: Reflections on Human Nature*. New York: Oxford University Press.

Cann, R.L. 2001. Genetic clues to dispersal in human populatons: Retracing the past from the present. *Science* 291:1742–1748.

Chalmers, D.J. 1996. *The Conscious Mind: In Search of a Fundamental Theory*. New York: Oxford University Press.

Chang, E.C. 2001. *Optimism and Pessimism: Implications for Theory, Research, and Practice*. Washington, D.C.: American Psychological Association.

Chomsky, N. 1972. *Language and Mind*. Enlarged ed. New York: Harcourt Brace Jovanovich.

Chomsky, N. 1980. *Rules and Representations*. New York: Columbia University Press.

Churchland, P.M. 1996. *The Engine of Reason, the Seat of the Soul*. Cambridge: MIT Press.

Ciarrochi, J., Forgas, J.P., & Mayer, J.D. (Eds.) 2001. *Emotional Intelligence in Everyday Life: A Scientific Inquiry.* Philadelphia: Psychology Press.

Cohen, G. 1996. *Memory in the Real World.* 2nd Ed. East Sussex: Psychology Press.

Cosgrove, G.R. 2000. Surgery for psychiatric disorders. *CNS Spectrums* 5 (10): 43–47.

Cousins, N. 1981. *Human Options.* New York: W.W. Norton.

Cousins, N. 1989. *Head First—The Biology of Hope.* New York: E.P. Dutton.

Couvalis, G. 1997. *The Philosophy of Science: Science and Objectivity.* London: Sage.

Craik, K.J.W. 1943. *The Nature of Explanation.* Cambridge: Cambridge University Press.

Crick, F. 1994. *The Astonishing Hypothesis: The Scientific Search for the Soul.* New York: Scribner.

Crook, J.H. 1980. *The Evolution of Human Consciousness.* Oxford: Clarendon Press.

Csikszentmihalyi, M. 1990. *Flow: The Psychology of Optimal Experience.* New York: Harper & Row.

Csikszentmihalyi, M. 1997. *Finding Flow: The Psychology of Engagement with Everyday Life.* New York: Basic Books.

Cullingford, C. 1999. *The Human Experience: The Early Years.* Aldershot: Ashgate Publishing.

Dalai Lama & Cutler, H.C. 1998. *The Art of Happiness: A Handbook for Living.* New York: Riverhead Books.

Damasio, A.R. 1994. *Descartes' Error: Emotion, Reason, and the Human Brain.* New York: G.P. Putnam's Sons.

Damasio, A.R. 1999. *The Feeling of What Happens: Body and Emotion in the Making of Consciousness.* New York: Harcourt Brace.

Darwin, C. 1872 (1934). *The Expression of the Emotions in Man and Animals.* Abridged ed. London: Watts.

Darwin, C. 1881. *The Descent of Man and Selection in Relation to Sex.* London: John Murray.

Davies, P. 1996. *About Time: Einstein's Unfinished Revolution.* New York: Simon & Schuster.

Dawes, R.M. 1988. *Rational Choice in an Uncertain World.* New York: Harcourt Brace Jovanovich.

Dawkins, R. 1976. *The Selfish Gene.* Oxford: Oxford University Press.

Day, J.P. 1991. *Hope: A Philosophical Inquiry.* Helsinki: Philosophical Society of Finland.

Deacon, T.W. 1997. *The Symbolic Species: The Co-Evolution of Language and the Brain.* New York: W.W. Norton.

Deckel, A.W., Hesselbrock, V., & Bauer L. 1996. Antisocial personality disorder, childhood delinquency, and frontal lobe functioning: EEG and neuropsychological findings. *Journal of Clinical Psychology* 52:639–650.

Dehaene, S. 1997. *The Number Sense: How the Mind Creates Mathematics.* New York: Oxford University Press.

Delbanco, A. 1999. *The Real American Dream: A Meditation on Hope.* Cambridge: Harvard University Press.

De Lys, C. 1957. *A Treasury of Superstitions.* New York: Gramercy Books.

Dennett, D.C. 1991. *Consciousness Explained*. Boston: Little Brown.

Dennett, D.C. 1996. *Kinds of Minds: Towards an Understanding of Consciousness*. New York: Basic Books.

De Sousa, R. 1987. *The Rationality of Emotion*. Cambridge: MIT Press.

Desroche, H. 1979. *The Sociology of Hope*. London: Routledge & Kegan Paul.

de Waal, F. 1996. *Good Natured: The Origins of Right and Wrong in Humans and Other Animals*. Cambridge: Harvard University Press.

Diamond, J. 1992. *The Third Chimpanzee: The Evolution and Future of the Human Animal*. New York: Harper Collins.

Diamond, J. 1997. *Guns, Germs, and Steel: The Fates of Human Societies*. New York: W.W. Norton.

Dobzhansky, T. 1962. *Mankind Evolving: The Evolution of the Human Species*. New Haven: Yale University Press.

Dretske, F. 1988. *Explaining Behavior: Reason in a World of Causes*. Cambridge: MIT Press.

Dreyfus, H.L. 1979. *What Computers Still Can't Do: A Critique of Artificial Reason*. Cambridge: MIT Press.

Dudai, Y. 1989. *The Neurobiology of Memory: Concept, Findings, Trends*. New York: Oxford University Press.

Dunn, J. 1988. *The Beginnings of Social Understanding*. Cambridge: Harvard University Press.

Eckblad, G. 1981. *Scheme Theory: A Conceptual Framework for Cognitive-Motivational Processes*. London: Academic Press.

Eckman, P. & Davidson, R.J. (Eds.) 1994. *The Nature of Emotion*. New York: Oxford University Press.

Edelman, G.M. 1987. *Neural Darwinism: The Theory of Neuronal Group Selection*. New York: Basic Books.

Edelman, G.M. 1992. *Bright Air, Brilliant Fire: On the Matter of the Mind*. New York: Basic Books.

Edelman, G.M. & Tononi, G. 2000. *A Universe of Consciousness: How Matter Becomes Imagination*. New York: Basic Books.

Ehrlich, P.R. 2000. *Human Natures: Genes, Cultures, and the Human Prospect*. Washington, D.C.: Island Press.

Einstein, A. 1954. *Ideas and Opinions*. New York: Crown.

Eiseley, L. 1946. *The Immense Journey*. New York: Vintage Books.

Emmons, R.A. 1999. *The Psychology of Ultimate Concerns: Motivation and Spirituality in Personality*. New York: Guilford Press.

Engel, G.L. 1961. Is grief a disease? A challenge for medical research. *Psychosomatic Medicine* 23:18–22.

Engel, G.L. & Schmale, A.H. 1972. Conservation-withdrawal: A primary regulatory process for organismic homeostasis. In R. Porter & J. Knight (Eds.), *Physiology, Emotion and Psychosomatic Illness*. Ciba Foundation Symposium 8. Amsterdam: Elsevier–Excerpta Medica.

Evans, D. 2001. *Emotion: The Science of Sentiment.* Oxford: Oxford University Press.

Farb, P. 1978. *Humankind.* Boston: Houghton Mifflin.

Farran, C.J., Herth, K.A., & Popovich, J.M. 1995. *Hope and Hopelessness.* Thousand Oaks: Sage Publications.

Fauconnier, G. & Turner, M. 2002. *The Way We Think: Conceptual Blending and the Mind's Hidden Complexities.* New York: Basic Books.

Feather, N.T. (Ed.) 1982. *Expectations and Actions: Expectation-Value Models in Psychology.* Hillsdale: Lawrence Erlbaum.

Feinman, G.M. & Manzanilla, L. 2000. *Cultural Evolution: Contemporary Viewpoints.* New York: Kluwer Academic/Plenum.

Feynman, R.P. 1998. *The Meaning of It All.* Reading: Addison-Wesley.

Flaherty, M.G. 1999. *A Watched Pot: How We Experience Time.* New York: New York University Press.

Foley, R. 1995. *Humans Before Humanity.* Oxford: Blackwell.

Foster, J.K. & Jelicic, M. 1999. *Memory: Systems, Process, or Function.* Oxford: Oxford University Press.

Frank, J. 1961. *Persuasion and Healing: A Comparative Study of Psychotherapy.* Baltimore: Johns Hopkins University Press.

Frankl, V.E. 1959. *Man's Search for Meaning: An Introduction to Logotherapy.* Boston: Beacon Press.

Franklin, J. 2001. *The Science of Conjecture: Evidence and Probability before Pascal.* Baltimore: Johns Hopkins University Press.

Fraser, J.T., Haber, F.C., & Muller, G.H. (Eds.) 1972. *The Study of Time.* Berlin: Springer-Verlag.

Frazer, J.G. 1950. *The Golden Bough: A Study in Magic and Religion.* Abridged ed. London: Macmillan.

Freud, A. 1946. *The Ego and Mechanisms of Defense.* New York: International Universities Press.

Freud, S. 1913 (1950). *Totem and Taboo: Some Points of Agreement between the Mentalities of Savages and Neurotics.* Trans. J. Strachey. London: Routledge & Kegan Paul.

Freud, S. 1917. Mourning and melancholia. In *General Psychological Theory: Papers on Metapsychology.* New York: Collier.

Freud, S. 1930 (1949). *Civilzation and Its Discontents.* London: Hogarth Press.

Freud, S. 1933 (1949). A philosophy of life: Lecture 35 in *New Introductory Lectures on Psychoanalysis,* 4th ed. London: Hogarth Press.

Friedman, W. 1990. *About Time: Inventing the Fourth Dimension.* Cambridge: MIT Press.

Frijda, N.H. 1986. *The Emotions.* Cambridge: Cambridge University Press.

Frijda, N.H. 1988. The laws of emotion. *American Psychologist* 43:349–358.

Fromm, E. 1968. *The Revolution of Hope: Towards a Humanized Technology.* New York: Harper & Row.

Fuller, R.B. 1973. *Intuition.* New York: Anchor Books.

Fuster, J.M. 1985. The prefrontal cortex, mediator of cross-temporal contingencies. *Human Neurobiology* 4:169–179.

Fuster, J.M. 1997. *The Prefrontal Cortex: Anatomy, Physiology, and Neuropsychology of the Frontal Lobe.* 3rd ed. Philadelphia: Lippincott-Raven.

Garbarino, J. 1988. *The Future: As If It Really Mattered.* Larchmont: Bookmakers Guild.

Garber, J. & Seligman, M.E.P. 1980. *Human Helplessness: Theory and Applications.* New York: Academic Press.

Gazzaniga, M.S. 1998. *The Mind's Past.* Berkeley: University of California Press.

Geertz, C. 1973. *The Interpretation of Cultures: Selected Essays.* New York: Basic Books.

Gell, A. 1992. *The Anthropology of Time: Cultural Constructions of Temporal Maps and Images.* Oxford: Berg.

Gentner, D., Holyoak, K.J., & Kokinov, B.N. (Eds.) 2001. *The Analogical Mind: Perspectives from Cognitive Science.* Cambridge: MIT Press.

Ghiglieari, M.P. 1999. *The Dark Side of Man: Tracing the Origins of Male Violence.* Reading: Perseus Books.

Gigerenzer, G. & Murray, D.J. 1987 *Cognition as Intuitive Statistics.* Hillsdale: Lawrence Erlbaum.

Goldman, M.S. 2002. Expectancy and risk for alcoholism: The unfortunate exploitation of a fundamental characteristic of neurobiological adaptation. *Alcohol Clinical and Experimental Research* 26 (5): 737–46.

Goldman-Rakic, P.S. 1984. The frontal lobes: Uncharted provinces of the brain. *Trends in Neuroscience* 7:425–429.

Goldsmith, T.H. 1991. *The Biological Roots of Human Nature: Forging Links between Evolution and Behavior.* New York: Oxford University Press.

Goleman, D. 1995. *Emotional Intelligence.* New York: Bantam Books.

Goodwin, F.K. & Jamison, K.R. 1990. *Manic Depressive Illness.* New York: Oxford University Press.

Gopnik, A. & Melzoff, A.N. 1996. *Words, Thoughts and Theories.* Cambridge: MIT Press.

Gopnik, A., Melzoff, A.N. & Kuhl, P.K. 1999. *The Scientist in the Crib: Minds, Brains, and How Children Learn.* New York: William Morrow.

Gorman, B.S. & Wessman, A.E. (Eds.) 1972. *The Personal Experience of Time.* New York: Plenum Press.

Gould, S.J. 1999. *Rock of Ages: Science and Religion in the Fullness of Life.* New York: Ballantine Publishing Group.

Graef, H. 1959. *Modern Gloom and Christian Hope.* Chicago: Henry Regnery.

Greenfield, S. 1995. *Journey to the Centers of the Mind: Toward a Science of Consciousness.* New York: W.H. Freeman.

Greenfield, S. 2000. *The Private Life of the Brain: Emotions, Consciousness, and the Secrets of the Self.* New York: John Wiley.

Greenspan, S.I. 1997. *The Growth of the Mind and the Endangered Origins of Intelligence.* Reading: Addison-Wesley.

Gregory. R. 1986. Minds, machines and meaning. In S. Rose & L. Appignanesi (Eds.), *Science and Beyond.* Oxford: Basil Blackwell.

Griffin, D.R. 1976. *The Question of Animal Awareness: Evolutionary Continuity of Mental Experience.* New York: Rockefeller University Press.

Griffin, D.R. 1984. *Animal Thinking.* Cambridge: Harvard University Press.

Haith, M.M. Benson, J.B., Roberts, R.J., Jr., & Pennington, B.F. (Eds.) 1994. *The Development of Future-Oriented Processes.* Chicago: University of Chicago Press.

Haldane, J.B.S. 1940. *Possible Worlds.* London: Evergreen Books.

Hall, E.T. 1983. *The Dance of Life: The Other Dimension of Time.* New York: Doubleday.

Hardin, G. 1968. The tragedy of the commons. *Science* 162:1243–1248.

Harris, J.C. 1995. *Developmental Neuropsychiatry.* New York: Oxford University Press.

Hass, H. 1970. *The Human Animal: The Mystery of Man's Behavior.* New York: G. P. Putnam's Sons.

Heidegger, M. 1924 (1992). *The Concept of Time.* Trans. W. McNeill. Oxford: Blackwell.

Heilbroner, R. 1995. *Visions of the Future.* New York: Oxford University Press.

Helfrich, H. (Ed.) 1996. *Time and Mind.* Seattle: Hogrefe & Huber.

Hellige, J.B. 1993. *Hemispheric Asymmetry: What's Right and What's Left.* Cambridge: Harvard University Press.

Hobson, J.A. 1999. *Consciousness.* New York: Scientific American Library.

Hoffman, M. 1997. *The NPR Classical Music Companion: Terms and Concepts from A to Z.* New York: Houghton Mifflin.

Holland, C.H. 1999. *The Idea of Time.* Chichester: John Wiley & Sons.

Horgan, J. 1999. *The Undiscovered Mind: How the Human Brain Defies Replication, Medication, and Explanation.* New York: Free Press.

Horney, K. 1939. *New Ways in Psychoanalysis.* New York: W.W. Norton.

Hughes, R. 1988. *The Fatal Shore.* New York: Vintage Books.

Hughes, R. 1993. *Culture of Complaint: The Fraying of America.* New York: Oxford University Press.

Hume, D. 1739 (1978). *A Treatise on Human Nature.* Oxford: Clarendon Press.

Humphrey, N. 1992. *A History of the Mind.* New York: Simon & Schuster.

Hundert, E.M. 1989 *Philosophy, Psychiatry and Neuroscience: Three Approaches to the Mind.* Oxford: Clarendon Press.

Hutschnecker, A.A. 1981. *Hope: The Dynamics of Self-Fulfillment.* New York: G.P. Putnam & Sons.

Ingvar, D.H. 1985. Memory of the future: An essay on the temporal organization of conscious awareness. *Human Neurobiology* 4:127–136.

Jackendoff, R. 1994. *Patterns in the Mind: Language and Human Nature.* New York: Basic Books.

James, W. 1890. *The Principles of Psychology.* New York: Henry Holt.

Jastrow, R. 1981. *The Enchanted Loom: Mind in the Universe.* New York: Simon & Schuster.

Jaynes, J. 1976. *The Origins of Consciousness in the Breakdown of the Bicameral Mind.* Boston: Houghton Mifflin.

Johnson, G. 1992. *In the Palaces of Memory: How We Build the Worlds Inside Our Heads.* New York: Vintage Books.

Johnson, J.G., Cohen P., Brown, J., Smailes, E.M., & Bernstein, D.P. 1999. Childhood maltreatment increases risk for personality disorders during early adulthood. *Archives of General Psychiatry* 56:600–608.

Johnson-Laird, P.N. 1983. *Mental Models: Towards a Cognitive Science of Language, Inference, and Consciousness.* Cambridge: Harvard University Press.

Johnston, V.S. 1999. *Why We Feel: The Science of Human Emotions.* Reading: Perseus Books.

Kagan, J. 1978. *The Growth of the Child: Reflections on Human Development.* New York: W.W. Norton.

Kagan, J. 1984. *The Nature of the Child.* New York: Basic Books.

Kagan, J. 1998. *Three Seductive Ideas.* Cambridge: Harvard University Press.

Kahneman, D. & Tversky, A. (Eds.) 2000. *Choices, Values, and Frames.* Cambridge: Cambridge Universiy Press.

Kandel, E.R., Schwartz, J.H., & Jessell, T.M. (Eds.) 2000. *Principles of Neural Science.* 4th ed. New York: McGraw-Hill.

Kant, I. 1781 (1963). *Critique of Pure Reason.* Trans. N.K. Smith. London: Macmillan.

Kelly, G.A. 1955. *The Psychology of Personal Constructs.* New York: W.W. Norton.

Kinget, G.M. 1987. *On Being Human.* Lanham: University Presses of America.

Kleinman, A. & Good, B. (Eds.) 1985. *Culture and Depression: Studies in the Anthropology and Cross-cultural Psychiatry of Affect and Disorder.* Berkeley: University of California Press.

Köhler, W. 1938. *The Place of Value in a World of Facts.* New York: Liveright.

Kramer, J.D. 1988. *The Time of Music: New Meanings, New Temporalities, New Listening Strategies.* New York: Schirmer Books.

Krasnegor, N.A., Lyon, G.R., & Goldman-Rakic, P.S. 1997. *Development of the Prefrontal Cortex: Evolution, Neurobiology, and Behavior.* Baltimore: Paul H. Brookes.

Kübler-Ross, E. 1969. *On Death and Dying.* Reprint ed. New York: Collier Books.

Kuhn, T.S. 1970. *The Structure of Scientific Revolutions.* 2nd ed. Chicago: University of Chicago Press.

Kuper, A. 1994. *The Chosen Primate: Human Nature and Cultural Diversity.* Cambridge: Harvard University Press.

Kushner, H. 1989. *When Bad Things Happen to Good People.* New York: Bonny V. Fetterman.

Lamb, K. & Lamb A. 1971. *Hope.* London: C.A. Watts.

Landman, J. 1993. *Regret: The Persistence of the Possible.* New York: Oxford University Press.

Langer, S.K. 1998. *Mind: An Essay on Human Feeling.* Baltimore: Johns Hopkins University Press.

Lasch, C. 1979. *The Culture of Narcissism: American Life in an Age of Diminishing Expectations.* New York: W.W. Norton.

Lazarus, R.S. & Lazarus, B.N. 1994. *Passion and Reason: Making Sense of Our Emotions..* New York: Oxford University Press.

Leakey, R. 1994. *The Origin of Humankind.* New York: Basic Books.

Le Bon, G. 1903. *The Crowd.* London: Fisher Unwin.

LeDoux, J. 1996. *The Emotional Brain: The Mysterious Underpinnings of Emotional Life.* New York: Simon & Schuster.

LeDoux, J. 2002. *Synaptic Self: How Our Brains Become Who We Are.* New York: Viking.

Lee, D. 1950. Codification of reality: Lineal and non-lineal. *Psychosomatic Medicine* 12:2.

Lens, W. & Moreas, M-A. 1994. Future time perspective: An individual and a societal approach. In Z. Zaleski (Ed.), *Psychology of Future Orientation.* Lubin: Towarzystwo Naukowe KUL.

Lewis, A. 1932, The experience of time in mental disorder. *Proceedings of the Royal Society of Medicine* 25:611–620.

Lewis, M. & Haviland-Jones, J.M. (Eds.) 2000. *Handbook of Emotions.* 2nd ed. New York: Guilford Press.

Lieberman, P. 1991. *Uniquely Human: The Evolution of Speech, Thought, and Selfless Behavior.* Cambridge: Harvard University Press.

Lockhardt, R.S., Craik, F.I.M., & Jacoby, L. 1976. Depth of processing recognition and recall. In J. Brown (Ed.), *Recall and Recognition.* London: John Wiley & Sons.

Loftus, E.F. 2000. Remembering what never happened. In E. Tulving (Ed.), *Memory, Consciousness and the Brain.* Philadelphia: Psychology Press.

Loftus, G.R. & Loftus, E.F. 1976. *Human Memory: The Processing of Information.* New York: Erlbaum Associates.

Lorenz, K. 1981. *The Foundations of Ethology.* New York: Springer-Verlag.

Loritz, D. 1999. *How the Brain Evolved Language.* New York: Oxford University Press.

Lynch, W.F. 1974. *Images of Hope: Imagination as Healer of the Hopeless.* Notre Dame: University of Notre Dame Press.

Lynn, S.J. & McConkey, K.M. 1998. *Truth in Memory.* New York: Guilford Press.

Lyons, W. 1980. *Emotion.* Cambridge: Cambridge University Press.

McCrone, J. 1991. *The Ape That Spoke.* New York: William Morrow.

McDougall, W. 1921. *An Introduction to Social Psychology.* Boston: John W. Luce.

McGhee, P.E. 1979. *Humor: Its Origins and Development.* San Francisco: W.H. Freeman.

McGinn, C. 1999. *The Mysterious Flame: Conscious Minds in a Material World.* New York: Basic Books.

McGuire, M. & Troisi, A. 1998. *Darwinian Psychiatry.* New York: Oxford University Press.

McHugh, P. & Slavney, P. 1998. *The Perspectives of Psychiatry.* 2nd. ed. Baltimore: Johns Hopkins University Press.

McKinney, W.T. 1988. *Models of Mental Disorders: A New Comparative Psychiatry.* New York: Plenum.

MacLean, P.D. 1990. *The Triune Brain in Evolution: Role in Paleocerebral Functions.* New York: Plenum Press.

McNaughton, N. 1989. *Biology and Emotion,* Cambridge: Cambridge University Press.

McShane, J. 1991. *Cognitive Development: An Information Processing Approach.* Oxford: Basil Blackwell.

Machiavelli, N. 1520 (1961). *The Prince.* Trans. G. Bull. London: Penguin.

Maddux, J.E. 1999. Expectancies and the social-cognitive perspective: Basic principles, processes, and variables. In I. Kirsch (Ed.), *How Expectancies Shape Experience.* Washington, D.C.: American Psychological Association.

Mandler, G. 1997. *Human Nature Explored.* New York: Oxford University Press.

Martin, L.L. & Clore, G.L. (Eds.). 2001. *Theories of Mood and Cognition: A User's Handbook.* Mahwah: Lawrence Erlbaum.

Maslow, A.H. 1970. *Motivation and Personality.* 2nd Ed. New York: Harper & Row.

Masson, J.M. & McCarthy, S. 1995. *When Elephants Weep: The Emotional Lives of Animals.* New York: Delacorte Press.

Masterpasqua, F. & Perna, P.A. (Eds.) 1997. *The Psychological Meaning of Chaos: Translating Theory into Practice.* Washington, D.C.: American Psychological Association.

Mayer, J.D. 2001. A field guide to emotional intelligence. In J. Ciarrochi, J.P Forgas, & J.D. Mayer (Eds.), *Emotional Intelligence in Everyday Life: A Scientific Inquiry.* Philadelphia: Psychology Press.

Mayne, T.J. & Bonanno, G.A. (Eds.) 2001. *Emotions: Current Issues and Future Directions.* New York: Guilford Press.

Medawar, P. 1972. *The Hope of Progress.* London: Methuen.

Medin, D.L. & Atran, S. 1999. *Folkbiology.* Cambridge: MIT Press.

Melges, F.T. 1982. *Time and the Inner Future.* New York: John Wiley & Sons.

Melges, F.T. 1990. Identity and Temporal Perspective. In R.A. Block (Ed.), *Cognitive Models of Psychological Time.* Hillsdale: Lawrence Erlbaum.

Melges, F.T. & Bowlby, J. 1969. Types of hopelessness in psychopathological process. *Archives of General Psychiatry* 20:690–699.

Menninger, K. 1959. Hope. *American Journal of Psychiatry* 116:482–491.

Merry, U. 1995. *Coping with Uncertainty: Insights from the New Sciences of Chaos, Self-Organization and Complexity.* Westport: Praeger.

Miller, G.A., Galanter, E., & Pribram, K.H. 1960. *Plans and the Structure of Behavior.* New York: Holt, Rinehart & Winston.

Minkowki, E. 1933 (1970). *Lived Time: Phenomenological and Psychopathic Studies.* Trans. N. Metzel. Evanston: Northwestern University Press.

Morgan, E. 1995. *The Descent of the Child: Human Evolution from a Different Perspective.* New York: Oxford University Press.

Morris, R. 1985. *Time's Arrows: Scientific Attitudes towards Time.* New York: Simon & Schuster.

Mountcastle, V.B. 1975. The view from within: Pathways to the study of perception. *Johns Hopkins Medical Journal* 136:109–31.

Murray, H.A. (Ed.) 1968. *Myth and Mythmaking.* Boston: Beacon Press.

Nesse, R.M. 1991. What good is feeling bad? *The Sciences* 31:30–37.

Nesse, R.M. 2000. Is depression an adaptation? *Archives of General Psychiatry* 57:14–20.

Nichols, H. 1891. The psychology of time. *American Journal of Psychology* 3:453–529.

Noble, W. & Davidson, I. 1996. *Human Evolution, Language and Mind.* Cambridge: Cambridge University Press.

Norman, D.A. 1988. *The Psychology of Everyday Things.* New York: Basic Books.

Norwich, K.H. 1993. *Information, Sensation, and Perception.* San Diego: Academic Press.

Novey, S. 1968. *The Second Look: The Reconstruction of Personal History in Psychiatry and Psycholoanalysis.* Baltimore: Johns Hopkins University Press.

Nussbaum, M.C. 2001. *Upheavals of Thought: The Intelligence of Emotions.* Cambridge: Cambridge University Press.

Oatley, K. 1992. *Best Laid Schemes: The Psychology of Emotions.* Cambridge: Cambridge University Press.

Obeyesekere, G. 1985. Depression, Buddhism, and the work of culture in Sri Lanka. In A. Kleinman & B. Good (Eds.), *Culture and Depression.* Berkeley: Unversity of California Press.

Offer, D., Kaiz, M., Howard, K.I., & Bennett, E.S. 2000. The altering of reported experiences. *Journal of the American Academy of Child and Adolescent Psychiatry* 39 (6): 735–742.

O'Keane, V. 2000. Evolving model of depression as an expression of multiple interacting risk factors. *British Journal of Psychiatry* 177:482–483.

Orme, J.E. 1969. *Time, Experience and Behavior.* London: Iliffe Books.

Ornstein, R. 1991. *The Evolution of Consciousness.* New York: Touchstone.

Ornstein, R. 1997. *On the Experience of Time.* Boulder: Westview Press.

Ornstein, R. & Ehrlich, P. 1989. *New World, New Mind: Moving towards Conscious Evolution.* New York: Doubleday.

Ortony, A., Clore, G.L., & Collins, A. 1988. *The Cognitive Structure of Emotions.* New York: Cambridge University Press.

Oyama, S. 2000. *The Ontogeny of Information: Developmental Systems and Evolution.* 2nd. ed. Durham: Duke University Press.

Paivio, A. 1986. *Mental Representations: A Dual Coding Approach.* Oxford: Oxford University Press.

Panksepp, J. 1998. *Affective Neuroscience: The Foundations of Human and Animal Emotions.* New York: Oxford University Press.

Parkes, C.M. 1972. *Bereavement: Studies of Grief in Adult Life.* New York: International Universities Press.

Penrose, R. 1994. *Shadows of the Mind: A Search for the Missing Science of Consciousness.* Oxford: Oxford University Press.

Perner, J. 1991. *Understanding the Representational Mind.* Cambridge: MIT Press.

Piaget, J. 1927 (1969). *The Child's Conception of Time.* New York: Basic Books.

Piaget, J. & Inhelder, B. 1969. *The Psychology of the Child.* Trans. H. Weaver. New York: Basic Books.

Picard, R.W. 1997. *Affective Computing.* Cambridge: MIT Press.

Pinker, S. 1994. *The Language Instinct: How the Mind Creates Language.* New York: William Morrow.

Pinker, S. 1997. *How the Mind Works.* New York: W.W. Norton.

Pinker, S. 1999. *Words and Rules: The Ingredients of Language.* New York: Basic Books.

Plotkin, H. 1994. *Darwin Machines and the Nature of Knowledge.* Cambridge: Harvard University Press.

Plutchik, R. 1980. *Emotions: A Psychoevolutionary Synthesis.* New York: Harper & Row.

Plutchik, R. 2001. The Nature of Emotions. *American Scientist* 89:344–350.

Poidevin, R.L. & MacBeath, M. (Eds.) 1993. *The Philosophy of Time*. Oxford: Oxford University Press.

Popper, K.R. 1935 (1959). *The Logic of Scientific Discovery*. 2nd. ed. New York: Basic Books

Popper, K.R. 1965. *Conjectures and Refutations: The Growth of Scientific Knowledge*. 2nd ed. New York: Basic Books.

Preuss, T.M. 2000. What's human about human behavior? In M.S. Gazzaninga (Ed.), *The New Cognitive Neurosciences*. 2nd. ed. Cambridge: MIT Press.

Price, D.D. & Barrell, J.J. 1999. Expectation and desire in pain and pain reduction. In I. Kirsch (Ed.), *How Expectancies Shape Experience*. Washington, D.C.: American Psychological Association.

Pullum, G.K. 1991. *The Great Eskimo Vocabulary Hoax, and Other Irreverent Essays on the Study of Language*. Chicago: University of Chicago Press.

Radner, D. & Radner M. 1989. *Animal Consciousness*. New York: Prometheus Books.

Raine, A., Buschbaum, M.S., & LaCase, L. 1997. Brain abnormalities in murderers indicated by positiron emission tomogaphy. *Biological Psychiatry* 42:495–508.

Raine, A., Lencz, T., Bihrle, S., LaCase, L., & Colletti, P. 2000. Reduced prefrontal gray matter volume and reduced autonomic activity in antisocial personality disorder. *Archives of General Psychiatry* 57:119–127.

Rappaport, H. 1990. *Marking Time*. New York: Simon & Schuster.

Reading, A.J. 1977. Illness and disease. *Medical Clinics of North America* 61:703–710.

Restak, R.M. 1994. *The Modular Brain: How New Discoveries in Neuroscience Are Answering Age-old Questions about Memory, Free Will, Consciousness, and Personal Identity*. New York: Simon & Schuster.

Restak, R.M. 1995. *Brainscapes: An Introduction to What Neuroscience Has Learned about the Structure, Function, and Abilities of the Brain*. New York: Hyperion.

Rice, A.K. 1965. *Learning for Leadership*. London: Tavistock Publications.

Richards, E.G. 1998. *Mapping Time: The Calendar and Its History*. Oxford: Oxford University Press.

Richter, C.P. 1957. On the phenomenon of sudden death in animals and man. *Psychosomatic Medicine* 19:191–198.

Rifkin, J. 1987. *Time Wars: The Primary Conflict in Human History*. New York: Simon & Schuster.

Ristau, C.A. 1991. *Cognitive Ethology: The Minds of Other Animals*. Hillsdale: Lawrence Erlbaum.

Rivett, P. 1972. *Principles of Model Building: The Construction of Models for Decision Analysis*. London: John Wiley & Sons.

Roediger, H.L., Buckner, R.L., & McDermott, K.B. 1999. Components of processing. In J.K. Foster & M. Jelicic (Eds.), *Memory: Systems, Process, or Function?* New York: Oxford University Press.

Rogers, L.J. 1997. *Minds of Their Own: Thinking and Awareness in Animals*. Sydney: Allen & Unwin.

Rogers, Y., Rutherford, A., & Bibby, P.A. (Eds.) 1992. *Models in the Mind: Theory, Perspective and Application*. London: Academic Press.

Rolston, H. 1987. *Science and Religion*. Philadelphia: Temple University Press.

Rose, S. 1992. *The Making of Memory: From Molecules to Mind*. New York: Doubleday.

Rotter, J. 1966. Generalized expectancies for internal versus external control of reinforcement. *Psychological Monographs* 80:1–28.

Russell, B. 1918 (1953). *Mysticism and Logic*. London: Penguin Books.

Russell, B. 1921. *The Analysis of Mind*. London: George Allen & Unwin.

Rutter, M. & Rutter, M. 1993. *Developing Minds: Challenge and Continuity Across the Life Span*. New York: Basic Books.

Rycroft, C. 1979. Steps to an ecology of hope. In R. Fitzgerald (Ed.), *The Sources of Hope*. Oxford: Permagon Press.

Ryff, C.D. & Singer, B.H. (Eds.) 2001. *Emotion, Social Relationships, and Health*. Oxford: Oxford University Press.

Ryle, G. 1949. *The Concept of Mind*. New York: Harper & Row.

Salk, J. 1972. *Man Unfolding*. New York: Harper & Row.

Sarewitz, D., Pielke, R.A., Jr., & Byerly, R., Jr. (Eds.). 2000. *Prediction: Science, Decision Making and the Future of Nature*. Washington, D.C.: Island Press.

Sartre, J-P. 1971. *Sketch for a Theory of the Emotions*. London: Methuen.

Schacter, D.L. 1996. *Searching for Memory: The Brain, the Mind, and the Past*. New York: Basic Books.

Schacter, D.L. 2001. *The Seven Sins of Memory: How the Mind Forgets and Remembers*. Boston: Houghton Mifflin.

Schacter, D.L. & Tulving, E. (Eds). 1994. *Memory Systems 1994*. Cambridge: MIT Press.

Schank, R.C. 1982. *Dynamic Memory: A Theory of Reminding and Learning in Computers and People*. New York: Cambridge University Press.

Scherer, K.R., Schorr, A.A., & Johnstone, T. 2001. *Appraisal Processes in Emotion: Theory, Methods, Research*. New York: Oxford University Press.

Schlesinger, A.M., Jr. 1949. *The Politics of Hope*. Boston: Houghton Mifflin.

Schmale, A.H. & Engel, G.E. 1975. The role of conservation-withdrawal in depressive reactions. In E.J. Anthony & T. Benedict (Eds.), *Depression and Human Existence*. New York: Little Brown.

Schumacher, E.R. 1973. *Small Is Beautiful: Economics as if People Mattered*. New York: Harper & Row.

Searle, J.R. 1992. *The Rediscovery of the Mind*. Cambridge: MIT Press.

Sebba, A. 1972. Time and the modern self: Descartes, Rousseau, Beckett. In J.T. Fraser, F.C. Haber, & G.H. Muller (Eds.), *The Study of Time*. Berlin: Springer-Verlag.

Seddon, K. 1987. *Time: A Philosophical Treatment*. London: Croom Helm.

Seligman, M.E.P. 1975. *Helplessness: On Depression, Development and Death*. San Francisco: W.H. Freeman.

Seligman, M.E.P. 1991. *Learned Optimism*. New York: A.A. Knopf.

Seligman, M.E.P. 2002. *Authentic Happiness*. New York: Free Press.

Service, E.R. 1962. *Primitive Social Organization: An Evolutionary Perspective*. New York: Random House.

Service, E.R. 1975. *Origins of the State and Civilization*. New York: W.W. Norton.

Shackle, G.L.S. 1962. *Expectation in Economics*. Cambridge: Cambridge University Press.

Shackle, G.L.S. 1967. *Time in Economics*. Amsterdam: North-Holland.

Shackle, G.L.S. 1990. Time, expectation and uncertainty in economics. In J.L. Ford (Ed.), *Selected Essays*. Aldershot: Edward Elgar.

Shallis, M. 1983. *On Time: An Investigation into Scientific Knowledge and Human Experience*. New York: Schocken.

Shapin, S. 1996. *The Scientific Revolution*. Chicago: University of Chicago Press.

Sharp, C. 1981. *The Economics of Time*. New York: John Wiley & Sons.

Shaw, G.L. 2000. *Keeping Mozart in Mind*. San Diego: Academic Press.

Shiller, R.J. 2000. *Irrational Exuberance*. Princeton: Princeton University Press.

Shostak, M. 1983. *Nisa: The Life and Words of a !Kung Woman*. New York: Vintage Books.

Sigel, I.E. (Ed.) 1999. *Development of Mental Representations: Theories and Applications*. Mahwah: Lawrence Erlbaum Associates.

Silver, A.A. & Hagin, R.A. 1990. *Disorders of Learning in Childhood*. New York: John Wiley & Sons.

Skinner, B.F. 1972. *Beyond Freedom and Dignity*. New York: Alfred A. Knopf.

Slife, B.D. 1993. *Time and Psychological Explanation*. Albany: State University of New York Press.

Smith, M. 1980. *Hope and History, An Exploration*. New York: Harper & Row.

Snyder, C.R. 1994. *The Psychology of Hope*. New York: Free Press.

Snyder, C.R. (Ed.) 2000. *Handbook of Hope*. San Diego: Academic Press.

Solomon, A. 2001. *The Noonday Demon: An Atlas of Depression*. New York: Scribner.

Solomon, R.C. 1976. *The Passions*. Notre Dame: Notre Dame University Press.

Solomon, R.C. 2000. The philosophy of emotions. In M. Lewis & J.M. Haviland-Jones (Eds.), *Handbook of Emotions*. 2nd ed. New York: Guilford Press.

Spiro, H. 1998. *The Power of Hope: A Doctor's Perspective*. New Haven: Yale University Press.

Spitz, R. 1946. Anaclitic depression. *The Psychoanalytic Study of the Child* 2:313–342.

Spradlin, W.W. & Porterfield, P.B. 1979. *Human Biosociology: From Cell to Culture*. New York: Springer-Verlag.

Squire, L.R. 1987. *Memory and Brain*. New York: Oxford University Press.

Squire, L.R. & Kandel, E.R. 1999. *Memory: From Mind to Molecules*. New York: Scientific American Library.

Standing, L. 1973. Remembering 10,000 pictures. *Quarterly Journal of Experimental Psychology* 25:207–222.

Sternsher, B. (Ed.) 1999. *Hope Restored: How the New Deal Worked in Town and Country*. Chicago: Ivan R. Dee.

Stewart, T.R. 2000. Uncertainty, judgment, and error in prediction. In D. Sarewitz, R.A. Pielke, Jr., & R. Byerly, Jr. (Eds.), *Prediction: Science, Decision Making and the Future of Nature*. Washington, D.C.: Island Press.

Stille, A. 2002. *The Future of the Past*. New York: Farrar, Straus & Giroux.

Stoddard, J., Raine, A., Bihrle, S., & Buchsbaum, M. 1996. Prefrontal dysfunction in murderers lacking psychosocial deficits. In A. Raine, P.A. Brennan, D.P. Farrington, & S.A. Mednick (Eds.), *Biological Bases of Violence*. New York: Plenum Press.

Storr, A. 1992. *Music and the Mind*. New York: Free Press.

Stotland, E. 1969. *The Psychology of Hope*. San Francisco: Jossey-Bass.

Struss, D.T. & Benson, D.F. 1986. *The Frontal Lobes*. New York: Raven Press.

Styron, W. 1990. *Darkness Visible: A Memoir of Madness*. New York: Random House.

Suppe, F. (Ed.) 1977. *The Structure of Scientific Theories*. Urbana: University of Illinois Press.

Tattersall, I. 1998. *Becoming Human: Evolution and Human Uniqueness*. New York: Harcourt Brace.

Thomas, D.A. 1995. *Music and the Origins of Language: Theories from the French Enlightenment*. Cambridge: Cambridge University Press.

Tiger, L. 1979. *Optimism: The Biology of Hope*. New York: Simon & Schuster.

Tinbergen, N. 1955. *The Study of Instinct*. London: Oxford University Press.

Toffler, A. 1970. *Future Shock*. New York: W.W. Norton.

Tomasello, M. 1999. *The Cultural Origins of Human Cognition*. Cambridge: Harvard University Press.

Toulmin, S. & Goodfield, J. 1965. *The Discovery of Time*. New York: Harper & Row.

Trefil, J. 1997. *Are We Unique? A Scientist Explores the Unparalleled Intelligence of the Human Mind*. New York: John Wiley & Sons.

Trehub, A. 1991. *The Cognitive Brain*. Cambridge: MIT Press.

Trivers, H. 1985. *The Rhythm of Being: A Study of Temporality*. New York: Philosophical Library.

Tulving, E. 1976. Ecphoric Processes in Recall and Recognition. In J. Brown (Ed.), *Recall and Recognition*. London: John Wiley & Sons.

Tulving, E. (Ed.) 2000. *Memory, Consciousness and the Brain*. Philadelphia: Psychology Press.

Tulving, E. & Craik, F.I.M. (Eds.) 2000. *The Oxford Handbook of Memory*. New York: Oxford University Press.

Tulving, E. & Donaldson, W. (Eds.) 1972. *Organization of Memory*. New York: Academic Press.

Tye, M. 1995. *Ten Problems of Consciousness: A Representation Theory of the Phenomenal Mind*. Cambridge: MIT Press.

Vauclair, J. 1996. *Animal Cognition: An Introduction to Modern Comparative Psychology*. Cambridge: Harvard University Press.

Veninga, R.L. 1985. *A Gift of Hope*. Boston: Little, Brown.

Viorst, J. 1986. *Necessary Losses*. New York: Ballantine Books.

Vygotsky, L.S. 1978. *Mind in Society: The Development of Higher Psychological Processes.* M. Cole (Ed.). Cambridge: Harvard University Press.

Wade, N. (Ed.) 1998. *The Science Times Book of the Brain.* New York: Lyons Press.

Walker, S. 1983. *Animal Thought.* London: Routledge & Kegan Paul.

Wallin, N.L., Merker, B., & Brown, S. (Eds.) 2000. *The Origins of Music.* Cambridge: MIT Press.

Wallis, R. 1968. *Time: Fourth Dimension of the Mind.* New York: Harcourt Brace.

Weber, E. 1999. *Apocalypses: Prophesies, Cults and Millennial Beliefs through the Ages.* Cambridge: Harvard University Press.

Weiskrantz, L. 1988. *Thought Without Language.* Oxford: Clarendon Press.

White, L., Tursky, B., & Schwartz, G. (Eds.) 1985. *Placebo: Theory, Research, and Mechanisms.* New York: Guilford Press.

Whitrow, G.J. 1972. *The Nature of Time.* New York: Holt, Rinehart & Wiston.

Whitrow, G.J. 1989. *Time in History: The Evolution of Our General Awareness of Time and Temporal Perspective.* New York: Oxford University Press.

Whybrow, P.C. 1997. *A Mood Apart: Depression, Mania, and Other Afflictions of the Self.* New York: Basic Books.

Wilkes, K.V. 1988. "_____, yishi, duh, um, and consciousness." In A.J. Marcel & E. Bisiach (Eds.), *Consciousness in Contemporary Science.* Oxford: Clarendon Press.

Wilson, E.O. 1975. *Sociobiology: The New Synthesis.* Cambridge: Belknap Press of Harvard University Press.

Wilson, E.O. 1978. *On Human Nature.* Cambridge: Harvard University Press.

Wilson, E.O. 1998. *Consilience: The Unity of Human Knowledge.* New York: Alfred A. Knopf.

Wolfgang, A. (Ed.) 1979. *Nonverbal Behavior: Applications and Cultural Implications.* New York: Academic Press.

Wrangham, R. & Peterson, D. 1996. *Demonic Males: Apes and the Origins of Human Violence.* Boston: Houghton Mifflin.

Wright, G. 1984. *Behavioral Decision Theory: An Introduction.* Beverly Hills: Sage Publications.

Wright, R. 1995. *The Moral Animal: Evolutionary Psychology and Everyday Life.* New York: Vintage Books.

Yaker, H., Osmond, H., & Cheek, F. (Eds.) 1971. *The Future of Time.* New York: Doubleday.

Yalom, I. 1980. *Existential Psychotherapy.* New York: Basic Books.

Yando, R., Seitz, V., & Zigler, E. 1978. *Imitation: A Developmental Perspective.* Hillsdale: L. Erlbaum Associates.

Zaleski, Z. 1994. Towards a psychology of the personal future. In Z. Zaleski (Ed.), *Psychology of Future Orientation.* Lubin: Towarzystwo Naukowe KUL.

Zimbardo, P.G. 1994. *Foreword.* In Z. Zaleski (Ed.), *Psychology of Future Orientation.* Lubin: Towarzystwo Naukowe KUL.

Index

Bickerton, D., 101, 103, 106–7, 162–63
Bihrle, S., 169
bipolar disorder, 158
Bowlby, J., 151, 156
brain: aging and, 57–58, 117; cerebral cortex, 38, 101; information processing in, 37–39; limbic system, 45–46, 81; nature, nurture, and, 109; neural systems of, 45–46, 108–9; overview of, 45–46; 167–69; plasticity of, 117; prefrontal area of, 46, 105, 167–69; size of, 96, 108–9
brainwashing, 73, 143
Brand, S., 22, 171
Brown, G. W., 156
Bruner, J., 84
Brunner, R. D., 146
Bruton, H. J., 125, 144
Buddhism, 157–58
Buschbaum, M. S., 169
Byrne, R., 162

Calne, D., 20–21, 84
Calvin, W. H., 28
Campbell, D., 85
capitalism, 125, 144–45
categorical thinking, 113
cause and effect relationship, 112–13, 136–37
cave paintings, 96, 106
cerebral cortex, 38, 101
certainty, 16–17
change and uncertainty, 147–48
children: acquisition of language by, 96–97, 104–5, 111–12; environment for, 114, 115, 165; free will and, 70; future-orientation and, 7; memory and, 55; prefrontal cortex damage in, 168–69; present-orientation and, 110–11, 149; representational model and, 27; sentient awareness and, 62; socialization and enculturation of, 116–17
Chomsky, N., 104
Churchill, Winston, 143
Churchland, P. M., 69
Ciarrochi, J., 79
cities, emergence of, 92
class: crime and, 149; present-orientation and, 7

classification: of emotion, 75–77; in internal representation system, 47
cognitive appraisal, 81–82
cognitive functioning, modes of, 84
cognitive psychology, 26, 181 n. 9
communication: through emotional expression, 82–83, 102–4
community: change and uncertainty in, 147–48; crime and punishment in, 148–49, 163; description of, 140–41; religion and, 92; shared belief system of, 30–31, 133, 140
complacency, 9–10
confidence: and prediction of future, 16–17
Confucian tradition, 8
consciousness: altered states of, 72–73; content of, 66–67; definition of, 60–61; free will and, 69–71; functions of, xii, 65–66; information-processing and, 64–66; mental illness and, 169–70; origins of, 95–97; sentience and, 60–64
construct, personal, 29–30
control, locus of, 21
Copernicus, Nicolaus, 95
creativity, 33, 69
Crick, F., 61
crime and punishment, 148–49, 163
Crook, J. H., 26
Csikszentmihalyi, M., 72–73
Cullingford, C., 112–13
cults, 73, 143
cultural evolution, 90–91, 93–95, 147
culture: belief system and, 30–31, 133, 140; depression and, 157–58; description of, 15, 93; as heritage, 89; nonverbal communication and, 102–3; representational model and, 27; transmission of, 106, 116–17
curiosity, 196 n. 5
current-state emotions: description of, 76; examples of, 151; physical expression of, 82; sensory information system and, 79–80
Cutler, H. C., 85

Dalai Lama, 85
Damasio, A. R., 61, 62, 74, 168–69